COULD IT BE INSULIN RESISTANCE?

For Anna, Ella and Oliver

COULD IT BE INSULIN RESISTANCE?

Hanna Purdy

Foreword by
Dr Jerry Thompson

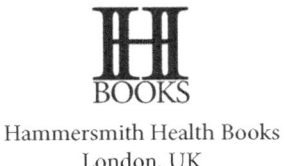

Hammersmith Health Books
London, UK

First published in 2020 by Hammersmith Health Books – an imprint of
Hammersmith Books Limited
4/4A Bloomsbury Square, London WC1A 2RP, UK
www.hammersmithbooks.co.uk

© 2020, Hanna Purdy

All rights reserved. No part of this publication may be reproduced, stored in any retrieval system or transmitted in any form or by any means, electronic, mechanical, photocopying, recording or otherwise, without the prior permission of the publishers and copyright holder.

The information contained in this book is for educational purposes only. It is the result of the study and the experience of the author. Whilst the information and advice offered are believed to be true and accurate at the time of going to press, neither the author nor the publisher can accept any legal responsibility or liability for any errors or omissions that may have been made or for any adverse effects which may occur as a result of following the recommendations given herein. Always consult a qualified medical practitioner if you have any concerns regarding your health.

British Library Cataloguing in Publication Data: A CIP record of this book is available from the British Library.

Print ISBN 978-1-78161-157-9
Ebook ISBN 978-1-78161-158-6

Commissioning editor: Georgina Bentliff
Designed and typeset by: Julie Bennett, Bespoke Publishing Ltd
Cover design by: Madeline Meckiffe
Index: Dr Laurence Errington
Production: Helen Whitehorn, Path Projects Ltd
Printed and bound by: TJ International Ltd, Cornwall, UK

Contents

About the Author — viii
Foreword — ix
Introduction — xi

1. What is insulin resistance? — 1
    Understanding your metabolism — 1
    Introducing insulin — 3
    What is hyperinsulinaemia? — 6
    Introducing mitochondria — 8
    Chronic inflammation as cause and effect — 10

2. What causes insulin resistance? — 15
    Sugar and starch — 16
    Advanced glycation end products (AGEs) — 18
    Alcohol — 19
    Refined oils — 20
    Eating too often — 22
    Chronic stress — 23
    Sleep problems — 24
    Unbalanced gut microbiome and leaky gut syndrome — 26
    Lack of exercise — 29
    Smoking and vaping — 30
    Summarising the causes of insulin resistance — 32

3. How do I know if I have insulin resistance? — 33
    Expanding waistline, weight gain and obesity — 36
    Hypoglycaemia – *low* blood sugar levels — 36
    Tiredness, low energy levels and mood swings — 37

Low immunity	37
Snoring and sleep apnoea	39
Problems with skin, including skin tags	39
Inner ear problems and tinnitus	40
Raised blood pressure	41
Cholesterol: low HDL cholesterol and high triglycerides	42
Summarising the signs and symptoms of insulin resistance	44
4. What are the consequences of insulin resistance?	**47**
Excess weight	47
Fatty liver	48
Hormone imbalance including polycystic ovary syndrome (PCOS)	51
Mouth and dental problems	53
Osteoporosis	54
Bowel problems	54
Chronic pain	56
Peripheral neuropathy	57
Gout	58
Type 2 diabetes	59
Heart disease	62
Cancer	63
Dementia and Alzheimer's disease	66
Eye problems: glaucoma and macular degeneration	68
Summarising the consequences of insulin resistance	70
5. How can I reverse insulin resistance?	**71**
Key actions	73
Eat a diet low in carbohydrates	74
Cut out sugar completely	77
Avoid starchy food	78
Avoid grains	79
Be careful with drinks	80
Don't eat too often	82
Eat only good quality, real food	85

Contents

Eat plenty of vegetables and herbs	86
Avoid most fruit, choose berries	87
Choose good quality protein, preferably organic	88
Avoid processed food	92
Choose natural fats and avoid refined oils and margarines	94
Keep your gut healthy	95
Exercise regularly	100
Learn to manage stress	102
Sleep well	106
6. Special considerations	**109**
Possible problems with a low-carbohydrate diet	109
Addictions and food cravings	111
What about calories?	112
Pregnancy and 'gestational diabetes'	112
Children and teenagers	114
Insulin resistance and the menopause	115
7. How do I eat to reverse insulin resistance?	**117**
Sample meals	117
Cost	118
Soups	119
Lunches	124
Dinners	134
Appendix	**155**
Low-, medium- and high-carbohydrate foods	155
The evidence	**157**
References	157
Other sources	177
Index	**207**

About the Author

Hanna Purdy is a Nurse Practitioner with specialisms in Public Health Nursing and Occupational Health nursing, currently working as an Urgent Care nurse in Cornwall, UK. Even in Urgent Care she finds daily evidence of the effects of insulin resistance and advises patients on lifestyle changes to reverse it and the symptoms they are so often suffering.

She is the mother of three happy, almost completely sugar-free teenagers who know all about, understand and live Hanna's approach to healthy eating. Her goal is to empower us all to recognise and overcome insulin resistance ourselves before it does us irreversible long-term damage.

Foreword

Few could have failed to witness the huge increase in obesity in our society over the last two decades, not least in our children. In parallel, we have seen a massive increase in diabetes, which now swallows up one-tenth of the NHS budget. Less well-known is the fact that fatty liver has increased rapidly and has now become the commonest chronic disease, affecting 20-30% of adults and, worryingly, up to 20% of children.

Hanna Purdy in her timely and well-researched book asks *Could it be Insulin Resistance?* Yes, it could be. In fact, it is the major underlying pathology behind all three of these mega problems and, as she explains, behind many other diseases as well. Never has insulin resistance been more important, and not just for those with disease but also for the seemingly healthy, especially those possessing a large belly.

Not only is insulin resistance important in itself but it is relatively straightforward to treat and Hanna does a first-class job explaining how to go about this. She includes a comprehensive discussion of what to eat and what not to eat. However, what often gets forgotten is *when not to eat* and this she covers brilliantly in the section 'Don't eat too often'. Understanding this section can make all the difference.

One thing I have noticed is, sooner or later, most patients have a blood test for lipids. This is done primarily for testing cholesterol but it can also diagnose insulin resistance. What few doctors realise is that insulin resistance is a far more useful predictor of disease than cholesterol, as Hanna explains, but sadly it receives less attention. Certainly if I were a patient I would be much more interested in my triglycerides and HDL (markers of insulin resistance) than my cholesterol.

Even if doctors do make this diagnosis, few would have the time to explain exactly what to do about it, but this book does just that.

Even for those familiar with insulin resistance there are surprises in this book. Hanna points out it can be implicated in snoring, in vertigo and tinnitus, in gout, in hypoglycaemia, in hormonal conditions such as thyroid disease and the menopause and in peripheral neuropathy. I suspect it is rarely tested for in these circumstances.

In obesity Hanna makes the point that it is almost impossible to lose weight if your insulin is consistently high. She rightly points out the pitfalls in treating type 2 diabetes with insulin which makes weight loss near impossible.

Finally, there is a useful section on possible problems when changing to a low-carbohydrate diet. I was unaware that extra salt was sometimes needed and sometimes extra water.

This is an excellent and much-needed book and if this knowledge were widely understood and put into action by the medical profession it would prevent an avalanche of disease, save the NHS millions of pounds and we would all be far healthier.

Dr Jerry Thompson
GP and Ecological doctor

Introduction

We are currently facing a crisis with chronic illness all over the world. It seems that the majority of adults and more and more children, teenagers and young adults are suffering from chronic symptoms that affect their everyday life. In the UK, where I am writing, the National Health Service (NHS) is battling under enormous pressure with the rising costs that these chronic problems lead to. Treating diabetes alone costs an estimated £14 billion a year, with 3.5 million people in the UK currently diagnosed with type 2 diabetes.[1] Many more are likely to be pre-diabetic and destined to face problems sooner or later. Over 9 million people in the UK are battling with musculoskeletal symptoms of some sort, many of them unable to work and often on long-term medication with difficult side-effects. Hundreds of thousands of people suffer from other types of chronic pain, with fibromyalgia alone estimated to affect 1.5 to 2 million people in the UK.[2] Fibromyalgia, a very complicated syndrome with chronic widespread pain, anxiety, depression and fatigue, seems to be getting increasingly common, with younger and younger sufferers.

Currently one in six people in the UK are suffering from a mental health problem.[3] Millions regularly take medication for conditions such as anxiety, depression and panic attacks. Cancer is also becoming more common. According to Cancer Research UK, one in two people will develop cancer at some point in their lives. The causes of cancer and the reasons for the increasing numbers of cases are still being debated, with the aging population being one of the proposed reasons. However, many scientists believe that there are other more significant reasons, with our lifestyle being the most likely factor in the development of cancer.[4, 5, 6]

The situation is more or less the same across many other countries. The Centers for Disease Control and Prevention (CDC) in the US publishes yearly Adult Obesity Prevalence Maps for 50 states in the US. According to them, more than 20% of adults in all states are now obese. In 2015-2016, over 93 million adults and 13.7 million children and young people in the US were reckoned to be obese.[7] At the same time, the number of obesity-related cancers is increasing and not only in the US, but around the world. The incidence of non-alcoholic fatty liver disease (NAFLD) is increasing rapidly and it is estimated that it will soon be the most likely indication for liver transplantation.[8, 9] According to a review published in 2018, 25% of adults worldwide suffer from NAFLD.[10] Many of the patients affected are still relatively young.

According to the World Health Organization (WHO), nearly 300 million people worldwide suffer from depression and 50 million from dementia. Nearly 18 million die each year from cardiovascular disease. These are very concerning figures.

The explosion in chronic disease is something I see every day in my current work as a nurse practitioner

Not only is the scale of these problems crippling the NHS here in the UK – something that affects everybody – but the suffering these conditions causes to individuals and their families is unimaginable… until it happens to you and yours. As I have said, the situation is the same in many parts of the world. We are all wondering why this is happening. In GPs' surgeries we can see the consequences of this problem every single day and it feels so overwhelming. I see this as a patient myself, but also as a

Introduction

registered nurse for over 20 years, and in my current work as a nurse practitioner treating many patients with these complicated symptoms. What can we do about all these symptoms? How can we help our patients?

To be able to answer those questions we need to understand the reasons why this is happening. Here, the most important thing to understand and remember is the fact that chronic conditions don't just happen, but are signs that **we are doing something wrong**. Almost always with any chronic symptom, there is something in our lifestyle causing it and all the associated suffering. When digging deeper, looking at common lifestyle issues, hearing from patients who have managed to find help for chronic conditions with lifestyle changes and, looking at many studies, it is obvious that one of the most important, if not the main, cause of all this suffering is the food we eat. To be more specific, the issue is processed food, sugar and excess carbohydrates, and the underlying problem they lead to – insulin resistance. There are other causes too for insulin resistance and we will look at all of these, but it seems that sugar and processed food, and the hormonal imbalance and inflammation they cause in our body, are the main reasons why many of us are so unwell.

One of the very first lessons I learned as a nurse in my anatomy and physiology course many years ago, was what an incredibly well organised and finely tuned system the human body is, not only in its functions, but also in its amazing ability to heal and repair itself in the right circumstances. To ensure all the functions necessary for life, a very fine balance must be maintained at all times all over the body. The wise practitioners of ancient Chinese and Indian medicine understood this. They continue to see illness as the result of a problem in this balance and know that to return the body's functioning back to health, it is important to look at the cause of this imbalance and change that. We seem to have forgotten this in our modern, Western medicine; instead of looking for the root of the problem, we try to treat the symptoms only and don't get very far.

We need to understand this point: that chronic symptoms are a result of an imbalance in the body and in many cases this is a hormonal imbalance caused by too much insulin. We cause this imbalance by eating the wrong foods, or by some other lifestyle issue, such as lack of sleep or other type of stress. The key to all this is to change our lifestyle; there is no medication to restore the balance. Our modern lifestyle sees many of us eating ultra-processed ready-made foods rather than following a natural diet. The most important problem is our intake of carbohydrates, and especially of sugar. We will be looking deeper into this issue to understand why it is a problem.

Chronic symptoms are very often the result of a hormonal imbalance caused by too much insulin

I am hoping to teach my readers, as I do my patients, the basics of how our metabolism works and why too much insulin can be a problem. We humans are naturally healthy; we are not meant to be chronically ill. Chronic illnesses and/or symptoms are not part of normal life or normal aging, and they don't 'just happen'. Instead of looking only for medication to suppress symptoms, we should always try to find their causes in our lifestyle and what we are doing generally, and to do something about them. We need to learn from our symptoms what it is that our body is trying to tell us and to work out what we can do to feel better. This way we can start to concentrate on our health instead of fighting our illnesses.

I know that many chronic illnesses are still often considered incurable and progressive, but this is very often not the case. As I have said, conditions such as type 2 diabetes are caused by lifestyle issues, so they can be reversed by lifestyle changes. There is no other cure, no magic pill to take; changes in lifestyle are

Introduction

necessary to reverse symptoms and restore health. Even when medical treatments are necessary in the presence of difficult illnesses, such as cancer, with lifestyle measures supporting the body during the illness, we are often much better prepared for the demands of the treatment, and are stronger, making the treatments much more likely to be successful.

When choosing the right food and drink, we are choosing to be healthy. Food is our medicine. In my work I have seen so many times how choosing the right food is the best start to improving all chronic health problems, all symptoms. Of course, we cannot always cure everything completely, but with proper nutrition it is always possible to significantly reduce the severity of any symptom. When our diet is the right one, often many other lifestyle factors automatically improve too. With proper nutritious 'fuel', we have more energy and endurance for our day. We find the will and time to exercise. It is also much easier to combat any dependencies, such as drinking, smoking or sugar addiction, when we eat right. Stress also is way more manageable with good food to give us more inner power. It is easier to stay positive.

The problem is, however, that many of us don't know what a healthy diet is and we are not aware of the huge problems caused, especially by sugar and excess carbohydrates. What should we eat in order to stay healthy and why is eating right often so difficult? One day we are told to eat this and another day that. To be able to understand what the healthy choices are, we need to know how the body works, how the food we eat is metabolised (processed in the body), how the hormones involved affect every single cell in our body and why this balance can go wrong.

Everyone has a physician inside him or her; we just have to help it in its work. The natural healing force within each one of us is the greatest force in getting well. Our food should be our medicine. Our medicine should be our food...

Hippocrates

Genes are often brought up when talking about chronic illnesses. Many believe that they are diabetic because it is 'in my genes' or likely to suffer from high blood pressure because it 'runs in the family'. It is of course true that genes do play a big part. Some of us are more prone to get cancer while others face heart disease as a result of a bad diet, for example. We are not all the same. Whatever illness is written in our genes, we can prevent it (in most cases) by turning off those genes, with proper nutrition and other lifestyle choices. Our DNA is not necessarily our destiny. The expression of our DNA can be turned off or on. This is what is called 'epigenetics'. Nutrients from our diet, especially, are a major source of epigenetic changes so food actually can change the way our genes behave even though we cannot change the sequence of our DNA.

Whatever illness is written in our genes, we can prevent it (in most cases) by turning off those genes

The information in this book is based on my own individual experience, and that of my family and friends, but also more widely on that of many of the patients I have seen and helped as a nurse. It is also based on some great books, articles and presentations I have come across while doing my research, and also many studies, available for anyone to read. I have included a list of many of these at the back of the book (page 177).

My aim is to give my readers tools to look after themselves properly, but because a book, being general, is not a good substitute for a face-to-face consultation with a doctor or nurse when battling with illness, I have to remind you to consult your health professional before making big changes, especially if you are taking medication.

Chapter 1

What is insulin resistance?

Understanding your metabolism

I am going to start with a simple explanation of how our metabolism works. By metabolism we mean all the different essential chemical reactions in the body that keep it functioning. These include the production of energy, for which we need fuel from food, and growth and repair, for which we need building blocks, also from our food. Energy and building blocks come from what we call 'macronutrients', the major proportion of our diet: protein, fats and carbohydrates. Carbohydrates consist of chains of sugars, such as glucose and fructose. Proteins are made of chains of amino acids. Fats consist of chains of fatty acids. Essential amino acids and essential fatty acids are those macronutrients we must get from our food as our bodies cannot make them. It is worth noting that there are no 'essential' carbohydrates.

There are no 'essential' carbohydrates

All these macronutrients – fat, protein and carbohydrates – are broken down by the body before being absorbed.

Carbohydrates and sugars

Carbohydrates/sugars and fat are the macronutrients mostly used as fuel for our metabolic reactions. Carbohydrates/sugars, are found mainly in plant-based foods: vegetables, fruit and grains. There are different types of sugars, including glucose, fructose and galactose. Fructose is naturally present in fruit and honey. Lactose is the sugar found in dairy products and is made up of two simpler sugars – glucose and galactose in equal amounts. Maltose is found in foods such as grains, and therefore in beer, and is made up of two glucose molecules. Starch in foods such as potatoes, bread and rice, consists of long chains of glucose molecules. Essentially then, all carbohydrates are sugars; when we eat carbohydrates, they are broken down into sugars for absorption. There are some differences in how these different sugars are handled by our body as we shall see in more detail below. In summary, glucose causes our blood sugar levels to rise immediately, stimulating the production of insulin. Fructose, on the other hand, is processed by the liver where it is converted mainly to glycogen for storage. There is no limitless storage space, however, and any excess fructose is converted into fat (a process known as *de novo* lipogenesis) in the liver.

Proteins and amino acids

Amino acids are used to grow, repair and rebuild cellular proteins in tissues all over our body, so essential amino acids are just that – essential. Proteins are also important in the production of different hormones and enzymes. Good sources of proteins are meat, poultry, fish and eggs, as well as some nuts and seeds. Animal-based foods contain all the essential amino acids, so they are known as 'complete' proteins. Plant-based foods don't – an important consideration for vegans when planning their meals.

Fats

Fats are important for energy but are also needed for cell growth and repair (the membranes surrounding every single cell are made of fat) and for hormone production. They are also essential for the absorption of fat-soluble vitamins (vitamins A, D and E). The fatty acids needed for these processes can be derived from natural sources such as butter, olive oil, fatty fish and meat, cheese, nuts and seeds. The metabolism of fat is different from that of carbohydrates and protein; the main difference is that it does not involve the hormone insulin.

Introducing insulin

Hormones are the body's chemical messengers, involved in all the physiological processes in the body, including metabolism and immune functions. There are many hormones that regulate our metabolism. These tell us whether we are hungry or full up and when to eat; they respond to the food we eat, burn it or store it. Of all these hormones, the main ones are insulin, glucagon, leptin and ghrelin. Ghrelin is a hunger hormone that causes us to feel hungry, thereby affecting our appetite and food intake. Leptin acts in just the opposite way: it stops feelings of hunger once the body's energy needs have been met. All of these hormones have very important roles, but here we will concentrate on insulin.

Insulin is produced by the beta cells in our pancreas. It regulates many metabolic processes that provide cells with essential energy. Its main function is to transfer sugar from the blood into the cells in muscles, liver and all other tissues, to be used in the production of ATP, the basic form of energy on which all our cells run. When we eat and our blood sugar (glucose) level rises, the pancreas responds by releasing insulin into our bloodstream to help transport the glucose into our cells.

Insulin is also involved in storing glucose as glycogen and fat. As I have said, any glucose that the cells don't need is stored away, by insulin. Insulin signals the liver but also the muscles and fat cells, to store this excess glucose for later use as glycogen (short term) and also as fat (longer term). Insulin also inhibits the use of these stores for energy. It prevents the breakdown of stored fat; when insulin levels are high, nothing will come out of storage. This is because if insulin is present, its opposite hormone – glucagon – is not released. As a result of the effects of insulin, our blood sugar levels return to normal after a meal, until we eat again. Between meals, when we don't eat, our insulin levels fall and as a result, glucagon is released. Glucagon prevents blood sugar levels from falling too low by stimulating the liver to break down stored sugar (glycogen) or stored fat, to be used for energy. There is naturally a good balance between insulin and glucagon and between eating and fasting. We either store food for energy when we eat, or burn it when we don't eat. Insulin and glucagon need to be in balance to keep blood glucose stable at an appropriate level.

When insulin levels are high, nothing will come out of storage

All of these hormones are very important, as is the carefully regulated balance of the whole endocrine (hormone) system. Any problems with one hormone affect other hormones and, in turn, the metabolic balance stops working the way it should. Insulin affects other hormones and, because it is a part of the body's energy 'feeding system', it is easy to understand how any problems with its proper functioning cause problems with other hormones too and with the whole metabolic system.

Table 1: The main functions of insulin and the effects of insulin resistance

Insulin function	How it works	What happens in insulin resistance
Maintains blood sugar levels	Insulin is acting like a key to all the cells for the glucose to enter, to be used as energy	Blood sugar levels remain elevated, the energy production in cells is affected

Chapter 1

Helps liver to store excess glucose	Insulin helps the liver to store excess glucose as glycogen for later use Insulin signals the liver to stop producing glucose when it is no longer needed	The glucose production in the liver might go out of control with the liver producing glucose even when it is not needed
Helps build up and maintain muscle mass	Insulin helps the muscle cells to store excess glucose as glycogen Insulin maintains muscle mass by stimulating the uptake of amino acids	Possible loss of muscle mass
Helps in fat metabolism	Insulin helps to store excess glucose as fat in the liver and fat cells when glycogen stores are full Insulin also inhibits the breakdown of fat in adipose tissue	Increased amounts of fat in fat tissue and the liver, which leads to excess weight and fatty liver. High insulin levels prevent fat from being broken down for energy
Maintains electrolyte balance	Insulin helps electrolytes such as potassium, magnesium and phosphate enter the cells	Electrolyte imbalance, water retention, raised blood pressure, worsening renal function
Insulin function has a direct effect on all hormones	Many functions of all of our hormones are linked to each other. Proper functioning of insulin is essential for overall hormonal balance. These hormones include thyroid hormones and insulin-like growth factors (IGFs) which help to control the secretion of growth hormone. They both stimulate cell growth and also have an important role in glucose metabolism	Problems with insulin lead to imbalance in other hormones, such as IGFs, cortisol, oestrogen and/or thyroid hormones, and vice versa. This can result in many problems, including excessive cell growth, oestrogen dominance and changes in thyroid function

To summarise insulin's key role of maintaining healthy blood sugar levels, the following continues in an ongoing chain:

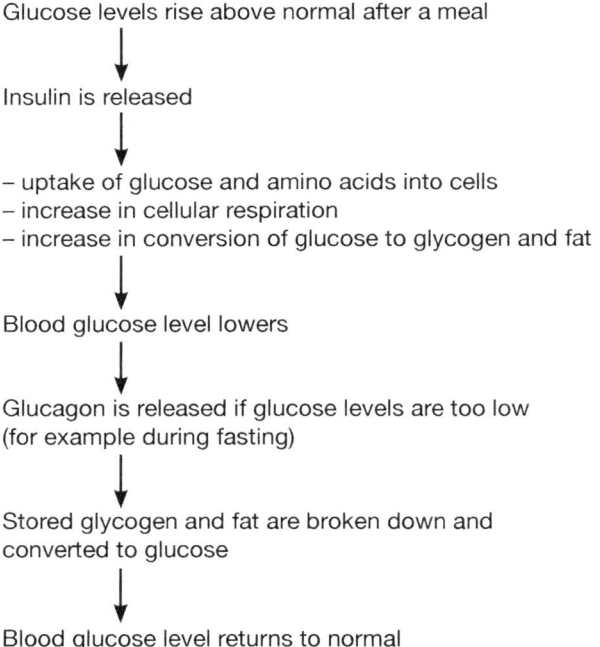

What is hyperinsulinaemia?

The biggest problem in keeping up a good metabolic balance is known to be having too much sugar (as sugar or carbohydrates) in our diet. In our modern diet we eat too much food mainly consisting of carbohydrates (sugar, as we have seen) and we eat too often. Insulin is needed almost all the time, not just in small amounts two or three times per day, and eventually our cells become resistant to its effects; they stop responding, possibly because of too much insulin in the body, or because the cells are already full of sugar and cannot take in any more. I will explain the reasons for the development of insulin resistance in more detail later in this book (see page 15).

Chapter 1

Insulin resistance describes the situation where the pancreas is producing what would normally be enough insulin but the cells are not responding to it as they did before and as they should. As a result, the body tries to compensate and so the pancreas has to produce even more insulin to achieve the same effect as before, to maintain normal blood sugar levels. This then leads to a situation where insulin levels in the body are constantly raised – this is what is known as hyperinsulinaemia. Unfortunately, with all this insulin in the body, the resistance also keeps getting worse. Eventually the body is no longer able to control blood sugar levels at all, which means that they stay above normal and so type 2 diabetes is diagnosed. However, insulin resistance is likely to have been present for many years, even decades, before this happens, causing many other problems.

If we eat too often, insulin is needed almost all the time

Insulin resistance and hyperinsulinaemia have many ill effects around the body. If we have insulin resistance, our cells' energy production system is unlikely to be working properly. In addition, we put on weight because insulin stores much of the glucose that can't get into cells to be metabolised in fat tissues and the liver. The amount of visceral fat – fat around our vital organs – increases, especially when there is excessive fat accumulating in the liver. Inflammation in the body increases, caused by constantly raised levels of insulin and sugar. Natural hormone balance in the body is disturbed. All of this causes many different symptoms and increases the risk of chronic diseases.

It is the raised levels of insulin initially that cause insulin resistance. As levels of insulin increase in the body, all tissues develop worsening resistance to its effects, including the liver. The liver itself has the ability to make glucose when needed. It is an important part of maintaining normal blood glucose levels by manufacturing glucose (a process called gluconeogenesis) and breaking down glycogen (glycogenolysis). In the presence of worsening insulin resistance, the liver stops producing glucose normally as insulin fails to suppress this production, but instead, glucose production can go out of control. In this situation, the liver produces more glucose even if blood glucose levels are already elevated. This leads to even more problems with blood glucose levels and even more insulin in the body. Insulin resistance itself leads to even worse hyperinsulinaemia, which again leads to even further resistance all over the body. The damaging cycle keeps getting worse and worse. This hormonal problem caused by high insulin levels is also known as **metabolic syndrome**.

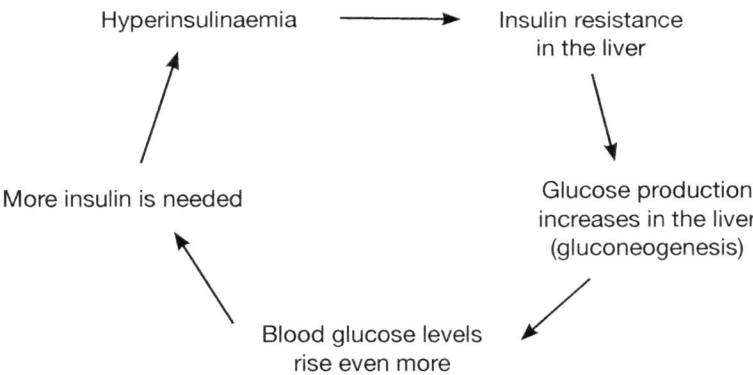

Introducing mitochondria

When looking more closely at our metabolism, we need to focus on our mitochondria. Mitochondria are organelles (sub-structures) in each cell that produce energy in the form of ATP (mentioned earlier), through the process of cellular respiration. For this they use acetate from carbohydrates or fat as fuel, with essential help from oxygen. Mitochondria also produce

Chapter 1

chemicals needed for other body functions, breaking down waste products and recycling them. Mitochondria are often referred to as the powerhouses of the cell because they generate ATP. This is essential for powering all the processes in our cells and therefore in our bodies.

The way mitochondria function is very complex and not fully understood, but we know that in addition to ATP production, they are also involved in other important processes such as apoptosis – planned cell death – and autophagy. **Apoptosis** happens naturally when the cell is damaged or no longer needed. This process is vital for growth and development, and it also works as a mechanism for the regulation of cell numbers and as a natural defence system for the removal of faulty cells. If apoptosis is not happening as it should, the result will be uncontrolled growth, a problem that can be seen in cancer, for example. **Autophagy** is the process whereby the cell recycles damaged and malfunctioning parts into new components. It is an important process of cellular cleansing when faulty cell contents are broken down and recycled for other purposes if apoptosis itself is not necessary. The cell thereby repairs itself. Problems causing cellular stress, such as nutrient deprivation and/or infections, can activate autophagy to keep our cells working, so it is again a vital function.

Our mitochondria make energy and look after the health of our cells but are highly susceptible to damage

Mitochondria are very dynamic, constantly dividing, changing shape and connecting and disconnecting to and from other mitochondria. There are different numbers of mitochondria in different tissues; the more energy is required, the higher the number. There are especially high numbers in tissues like the heart, brain and liver. Science has found that the more mitochondria we have in our cells and the better their function, the healthier we will be and the longer we will live. However, mitochondria are very susceptible to damage and dysfunction, and this damage contributes to both normal aging and to chronic symptoms and illnesses.

For proper mitochondrial function we need oxygen and many essential micronutrients (vitamins, minerals, polyphenols etc) from our diet. A diet low in micronutrients is therefore very harmful for mitochondrial functioning and other cellular processes. Insulin resistance is also very damaging. Mitochondrial function in diabetics, for example, is a lot poorer than in healthy people. Some studies also suggest that people suffering from type 2 diabetes have many fewer mitochondria than do people with a healthy metabolism.[1,2]

Chronic inflammation as cause and effect

Chronic inflammation is a problem we will talk about throughout this book. If you have insulin resistance you will also have chronic inflammation – it is both a cause and an effect in an ongoing vicious cycle. The development of insulin resistance activates many proinflammatory factors, causing oxidative stress and problems in normal metabolic functioning. Chronic inflammation is a situation where the body's normal immune system's responses to acute injury, or infection, linger on, leaving the body in a prolonged state of immunological alert, even when there is no acute infection or injury present. This can have long-term effects on the body and lead to tissue damage, which contributes to the development of many chronic illnesses. Chronic low-grade inflammation can have many causes including hidden dental infection and/or gum disease (page 53). Also, you are no doubt aware that recent research has shown a diet high in refined carbohydrates and especially sugar, is highly inflammatory.

Other causes of inflammation include refined and damaged vegetable oils, alcohol and smoking. It seems more research is needed to understand all the consequences of chronic inflammation but it is known to play a central part in many chronic illnesses. This is because these constant inflammatory responses in the body eventually damage healthy cells, tissues and organs. One example is damage to the endothelium (lining) of the arteries, which leads to atherosclerosis, a buildup of plaque in the arteries.

Chronic inflammation and insulin resistance go hand in hand

It is important to understand the problems chronic inflammation causes as it goes hand in hand with insulin resistance. Insulin resistance arises from inflammation and is thought to be one of the major causes of chronic inflammation in the body.

Chronic inflammation has a direct effect on the functioning of our mitochondria. Mitochondria are very important in inflammatory and immune cell functions. Studies have found that during inflammation, energy production by mitochondria drops to enable them to produce toxic compounds to increase the inflammation process further,[3,4,5] an important element in the body's defence system in acute situations but of course a problem when long-term, low-grade chronic inflammation is present. This process involves increased production of compounds called **'reactive oxygen species'** (ROS) by mitochondria, which damage cell structures. ROSs are produced in mitochondria as a byproduct of normal energy production anyway, and this is what is thought to be behind normal aging processes. The bigger the production of ROSs, however, the faster cellular damage and aging occur and the more chronic symptoms we have. This process is known as **'oxidative stress'**.

In addition, hormone functions being in balance affects how well our mitochondria keep working. An increase in glucagon (the opposite hormone to insulin, remember), stimulates the process of autophagy, for example, whereas glucose and insulin cause this cleaning up process to stop. Balance is very important here also – too much of either causes problems. We are not meant to eat all the time, but there has to be a balance between when we eat and collect all the nutrients we need and when we fast and clean our cells.

> *There has to be a balance between when we eat and collect all the nutrients we need and when we fast and clean our cells*

As mentioned earlier, when we get older, our mitochondrial functioning declines naturally. This means that the older we are, the more we have to look after our mitochondria. The speed of these aging changes can be increased greatly, not only by the wrong diet but also by lack of exercise and sleep, smoking and/or stress, all of which have been known to weaken mitochondrial function. Furthermore, some medications have a damaging effect on our mitochondria; examples include some anti-inflammatory drugs, statins, antidepressants and some antibiotics. As a nurse of many years' experience, I am pretty sure short-term medication is safe, but long-term is a different story. This is an example of why lifestyle measures are so important, instead of relying on long-term medication.

> *Insulin resistance is one of the biggest causes of the mitochondrial damage involved in many chronic diseases*

Mitochondrial dysfunction or damage can have many signs and symptoms in different organs. Tiredness and low energy levels, for example, might be signs of problems with energy production at the cellular level, in mitochondria. Chronic muscular pain

Chapter 1

could be a sign of damage to the mitochondria in the muscles. The more energy-demanding the tissue, the more mitochondria will be present, as I have said, and the more problems mitochondrial dysfunction will cause. As insulin resistance is one of the biggest causes of the mitochondrial damage involved in many chronic illnesses, many chronic symptoms are signs of problems in the mitochondria at cellular level. I talk more about the symptoms of insulin resistance in Chapter 3.

Chapter 2

What causes insulin resistance?

Insulin resistance is thought to be a protective mechanism in the main; our cells and organs are protecting themselves against a constant overload of glucose with which they cannot cope. They are already full of sugar and cannot take any more in. Also, as a result of too much glucose in the blood too often, insulin is present all the time. Just as in the development of any resistance, too much of something too often leads to increasing resistance. Insulin as a hormone is meant to be in the bloodstream only for short periods, not all the time. As the resistance of the cells to the effects of insulin keeps increasing, the body tries to compensate by increasing the amount of insulin even further, leading to chronic hyperinsulinaemia. As a result of hyperinsulinaemia, insulin resistance keeps getting worse. This development leads to chronic inflammation, which damages mitochondria in the cells of many tissues as discussed earlier. This is the root cause of many symptoms.

There are many reasons for this chain of events. Too much carbohydrate (sugar and starch) in the diet is the most important, but other lifestyle problems make the situation worse, such as alcohol, refined oils, eating too often, chronic stress, unbalanced gut microbiome, lack of exercise and smoking.

Starch and sugar

As discussed in Chapter 1, there are many different types of sugar. Some of them are found naturally in many foods whereas others are created artificially and added to processed foods.

Glucose is the main sugar used by every cell in our body for energy. As previously explained, glucose can also be stored in our body, mainly as glycogen in the liver and muscles, and it can be turned back into glucose if more energy is needed. Starchy foods like potatoes, grains, corn and rice are broken down in the body into glucose. The more we eat these foods during the day, the more sugar is absorbed into our bloodstream. When we talk about blood sugar levels, we mean blood *glucose* levels. Fructose is a type of sugar found naturally in fruit and berries. The body cannot use fructose directly; it is metabolised primarily by the liver. Both glucose and fructose are called 'monosaccharides'; they are made up of single sugar molecules of one type only. Some sugars are called 'disaccharides' as they contain two different types sugars and they cannot be absorbed by our bodies directly but have to be broken down into glucose and/or fructose/galactose molecules first.

Ordinary sugar, or 'table sugar', that we use in cooking or baking is called sucrose. Sucrose is made up of 50% glucose and 50% fructose. Some manufactured sugar syrups, such as high-fructose corn syrup, contain a higher proportion of fructose compared with glucose, but still have both sugars in them. As explained before, lactose is a type of sugar found in milk and other dairy products. Lactose is made up of two monosaccharides – glucose and galactose. Maltose is a type of sugar found in potatoes, corn, bread, pasta and beer; it is made up of glucose molecules.

Compared with glucose, fructose does not significantly raise blood sugar levels. For this reason it was considered to be a healthier option in the past and many products containing fructose were marketed to diabetics who needed to avoid ordinary sugar. However, studies have found the opposite to be true: fructose has turned out to be far worse than glucose when consumed in large amounts and it plays an important part in the development of insulin resistance. This is why table sugar and other sweeteners containing fructose are particularly problematic. As I have said, fructose is metabolised almost entirely in the liver, which can convert it into glucose for immediate use or glycogen for short-term storage, but also into triglycerides (composed of three fat molecules plus glycerol) if there is an excessive amount. Some of the fat stays in the liver, leading over time to a condition called fatty liver disease that is now recognised as widespread. This again makes insulin resistance worse, possibly because of inflammation in the liver as a result of stored fat, but also because of scarring (fibrosis) which decreases the sensitivity of the liver cells to insulin even further.

The more fructose is consumed, just as with alcohol, the more pressure there is on the liver, and the more likely the liver is to be damaged.

The metabolism of fructose is actually similar to that of alcohol, which explains why excess consumption of either causes fatty liver disease. We have only very limited capacity to metabolise fructose, just like alcohol, and any excess causes problems. You have to remember that even children these days are diagnosed with fatty liver because of sugar consumption. Parents don't know or think about the effects of sugar from this point of view. Most of us would never let our children consume alcohol but we don't realise that we allow similar damage to develop by letting them eat lots of sweets and other sugary foods or drinks, often every day.

Starchy foods cause lots of problems because they contain high amounts of carbohydrates that are composed of sugars and we eat too much of them. It is unfortunately quite normal to start the day with a carbohydrate-loaded breakfast with muesli or cereal, and/or bread/toast together with fruit juice, for example. Many people eat sandwiches for lunch, often with crisps and different snack bars. The most common family staple meals nearly always contain starchy foods like pasta, potatoes and rice. This breaks down to a lot of sugar. For example, according to the calculations of the Public Health Collaboration, if we have a bowl of bran flakes with milk, a slice of brown toast and a glass of apple juice for breakfast, we have digested 15-16 teaspoons of sugar just over one meal. This exceeds the World Health Organization's (WHO) daily sugar maximum recommendation of 6 teaspoons (approximately 25 grams).

Even when much of this sugar can be burned for energy throughout the body, especially if we are physically very active, it is still too much for most of us and we end up suffering from insulin resistance. We need to remember that all carbohydrates have this effect. Bread, for example, is a carbohydrate and it is important to understand that it does not matter whether we eat brown, white or wholegrain bread – all of them break down to sugar.

Advanced glycation end products (AGEs)

When we eat highly processed food, composed mainly of carbohydrates and sugar together with protein, and especially if this food has been cooked at a high temperature (in a deep-fat fryer, for example), the sugar in the food binds to the proteins or lipids in a process called glycation, forming 'advanced glycation end products' (AGEs). AGEs are harmful; amongst other problems, they trigger inflammatory responses in mitochondria in many organs, potentially leading to mitochondrial dysfunction and damage, as explained in Chapter 1.

AGEs are not formed only when we eat food cooked this way, but are also formed in the body when high levels of sugar are present in our blood (in type 2 diabetes). The sugar combines together with protein in the same way, through glycation reactions. We can measure these processes with HbA1C blood tests, for example. You may have had one or more of these if you are thought possibly to have diabetes type 2 – the test measures how much glucose has stuck on to the haemoglobin in your red blood cells, which indicates how well controlled your blood sugar levels have been over the past two to three months, something a single blood sugar test can't do.

These processes don't happen only in our blood, but in all other organs too. AGEs play a very important part in the development of diabetic complications, such as retinopathy, nephropathy, neuropathy and cardiomyopathy. Fructose is much more effective in forming AGEs than glucose, so avoiding table sugar (50% fructose) or other sweeteners containing high levels of fructose especially, is particularly important for people with diabetes.

Alcohol

Most of us are aware of how harmful excessive amounts of alcohol are. Like fructose, alcohol is metabolised mostly in the liver, putting pressure on this hard-working organ. This again leads to fatty liver. When there is too much fat in the liver, as explained previously, the situation may lead to inflammation and insulin resistance. Insulin resistance is common in people with alcohol-related liver problems, and insulin resistance increases the risk of more severe alcohol-related liver problems. It is important to remember that it is possible, and actually also quite common, to have a fatty liver even if body weight is normal.

There are also toxic byproducts produced in the liver when processing alcohol, such as acetaldehyde, as well as free radicals, all of which contribute to liver damage. Some studies have found that chronic drinking can also cause damage to the insulin-producing beta-cells in the pancreas. Of course, the effects of alcohol, like sugar, on existing insulin resistance vary and depend on how much we drink or our pattern of drinking. Certain alcoholic drinks, especially beer, also contain too much carbohydrate so are not advisable for anyone suffering from insulin resistance. Beer is more or less liquid bread.

Refined oils

As discussed earlier (page 2), fat is an essential part of our diet. We need saturated fats (SFAs) – solid fats found for example in butter, cheese, lard and coconut oil – for energy. Monounsaturated fats (MUFAs – omega-7 or -9 fatty acids, for example) which we can get from olive oil, various nuts and avocados, are not essential (we can make them for ourselves) but beneficial – for example, a study published in 2004 found that a diet high in omega-9 fatty acids may improve sensitivity to insulin.[1,2] We get polyunsaturated fats (PUFAs) mostly from nuts, seeds, oily fish and grass-fed meat. There are two types that are known to be essential – we cannot make them for ourselves – omega-3 and omega-6 fatty acids.

Omega-3 fatty acids are found mainly in fatty fish, free range eggs, hemp and chia seeds, seaweed and algae and also in meat and dairy products from *grass-fed* animals. There are three main forms: the first two are eicosapentaenoic acid (EPA) and docosahexaenoic acid (DHA), mostly in fish and seafood. These fatty acids are considered extremely healthy, especially for the brain, heart health and to reduce inflammation. The third type is called alpha-linolenic acid (ALA) which is mostly found in rapeseed oil, linseeds and hemp seeds as well as some nuts, especially walnuts. The body converts some ALA into EPA and DHA, but only to a very limited extent, which is why I do recommend eating non-farmed oily fish if at all possible.

Omega-3 fatty acids are a crucial part of cell membranes and also of the myelin sheaf that surrounds nerve cell fibres.

They are also the precursors (starter building blocks) for anti-inflammatory eicosanoids – biochemicals that help to switch off the inflammatory reaction to injury and infection once it is no longer needed.

Omega-6 fatty acids (mainly linoleic acid – LA) are found particularly in nuts and seeds, including sunflower seed, starflower and corn oils. There are also large amounts in processed food, usually as processed refined oils, though these have often been damaged by processing – see below. Omega-6 fatty acids are also essential constituents of our cell membranes but are precursors to pro-inflammatory eicosanoids, essential in the initial inflammatory response to injury and infection.

Both omega-3 and omega-6 fatty acids are essential, as I have said, and can be obtained only from our diet. They also need to be in the right balance; it seems we need more or less equal amounts of both though there is disagreement over this, with many guidelines recommending a ratio of 4 x omega-6 to 1 x omega-3. One of the problems in our modern diet is that it contains way too much omega-6 relative to omega-3. Instead of the ideal ratio, the estimated average ratio today is thought to be 16:1, because of the consumptions of processed food and vegetable oils. According to some studies, high omega-6 content in food may lead to chronic inflammation, especially if the omega-3 intake at the same time is low.[2, 3, 4, 5, 6, 7, 8] It has been shown that omega-3 fatty acids, especially DHA and EPA, can reduce existing inflammation and should be actively included in our diet.

Many vegetable and seed oils are highly unstable and when processed or heated form harmful aldehydes

The biggest problem with many vegetable and seed oils is that they are highly processed but also very unstable oils, relative to saturated fats, and known to form harmful compounds, called aldehydes, when heated to high temperatures. Chips cooked in beef dripping in the old-fashioned way do not contain high levels of aldehydes but because of the significantly lower price of refined vegetable oils, they are widely used in food manufacturing.

To stay healthy, we need to think about preventing or reducing chronic inflammation in our body. This means avoiding sugar and excessive insulin production, as already explained, but also avoiding other foods that are likely to cause inflammation. Such foods include refined, processed oils. As explained previously, insulin resistance promotes chronic inflammation, and many other factors, such as refined vegetable oils, increase this inflammation, leading to further escalation of insulin resistance and the development of its complications.

To support health and reduce inflammation in the body, in addition to fish and other seafood, I always recommend including extra-virgin olive oil in the diet. As explained above, oleic acid, a type of monounsaturated fatty acid that is the main constituent of olive oil, has many known health benefits.[9, 10, 11, 12, 13]

Eating too often

As previously explained, our hormones tell us whether we are hungry or full up, when to eat, and how to respond to the food we eat, by either burning it or storing it. With regard to eating, our bodies effectively work in two states: when we eat, the energy in our food is ingested and used or stored away for later use. When we are not eating, our bodies start to burn energy that has been stored as there is no more coming from food. These states need to be in good balance, like everything else.

If we eat too much carbohydrate too often, we will have too much insulin in our system <u>all the time</u>

If we are constantly eating every few hours, there is no balance. It was previously believed that to maintain steady blood sugar levels, we must not go without food for too long, but it was important to eat little and often by including snacks between main meals throughout the day. However, this way we are not letting our body rest and burn the stored energy. It is not good to eat more than three meals a day for this reason. If we eat all the time, and especially if we eat too much carbohydrate too often, we will have too much insulin in our system all the time. Don't forget, insulin is a hormone which stores the excess sugar as fat. It prevents the opposite hormone, glucagon, from working and so any burning of stored fat is impossible. This is the reason we often find it very difficult to lose weight – we are not allowing the 'not eating' phase to occur.

Chronic stress

It is very important to include stress in the long list of insulin-resistance-related problems and causes because, just like the food we consume, stress deeply affects every aspect of our health and can cause chronic health problems or make existing conditions much worse. It can also prevent us recovering even when all other lifestyle factors are in balance.

High stress levels are known to exacerbate insulin resistance and increase the risk of chronic illness. There are many reasons for this. One is that chronic stress is known to lead to problems with the micro-organisms in our gut. We will discuss this in further detail later (see 'microbiome', page 26). Another is the hormonal imbalance stress can cause. If the body is constantly releasing too much of the so-called 'stress hormones' – adrenalin and cortisol – as a result of chronic stress, these can affect insulin and other hormones; in this way, the overall hormone balance is affected. These stress hormones cause certain effects in our whole body which are beneficial in acute situations of possible danger ahead (we have all heard of the fight-or-flight response). These include raised heart rate and blood pressure as well as increased blood glucose, altered immune system responses and changes in the functioning of the digestive system. These useful responses in acute situations become a problem when the stress-related alarm is ongoing – we barely have enough to pay the rent, our boss is a bully, etc. Our immune system is suppressed because of the stress response being active instead; our ability to digest food properly is disrupted and the constant raised levels of stress hormones interfere with insulin, potentially lowering our insulin sensitivity, leading to the development or worsening of existing insulin resistance.

Chronic high levels of stress hormones can suppress our immune response, disrupt our digestion and lower our sensitivity to insulin

Of course, stress, and especially stress caused by factors and events in life we have no control over, can be extremely difficult to cope with, but it is important even in these situations to try to incorporate good stress management measures into everyday life to reduce the ill effects of chronic stress.

Sleep problems

Good sleep is extremely important for our health. We rest and our body cleans and repairs itself at a cellular level. We need this for our immune and metabolic functions too. Poor sleep, like stress, has a big impact on our health, including our metabolic health.

As you no doubt know, our natural sleep–wake rhythm is called our circadian rhythm. A number of hormones are involved in regulating this, including melatonin, growth hormone, thyroid stimulating hormone (TSH), cortisol, ghrelin and leptin.

Chapter 2

Hormone imbalance can therefore affect our sleep, and poor sleep can affect our overall hormone balance. Some of these hormones regulate our appetite, making us eat more and possibly crave unhealthy foods more if not in balance. Most importantly, sleep disturbances are a known risk factor for insulin resistance as they cause problems with insulin signaling and glucose metabolism. This is because stress levels rise as a result of poor sleep, upping levels of cortisol. Sleeping well really is important – the deep stage of sleep especially for blood sugar regulation and insulin sensitivity.

Sleep disturbances are a known risk factor for insulin resistance, causing problems with insulin signaling and glucose metabolism

Poor sleep may also affect our gut microbiome health (discussed next) and cause inflammation through stress. On the other hand, if our microbiome is not in good condition, our sleep is affected. This is because the sleep hormone melatonin is produced in our gut, as well as in the brain. Melatonin has an important role in our circadian rhythm, which regulates not only our sleep–wake cycle but also our glucose metabolism. Therefore, changes in melatonin production can make insulin resistance worse.

Sleep apnoea

As a reader of this book seeking information about insulin resistance, you may also have sleep apnoea. Many people suffering from insulin resistance also suffer from sleep apnoea, which interrupts their sleep even further. A night's sleep with sleep apnoea is usually poor because of chronic wakefulness and poor oxygen absorption and this causes tiredness during the day, leading to raised stress levels.

Unbalanced gut microbiome and leaky gut syndrome

Our gut microbiome (or 'gut flora'/'gut microbiota') is the collective term for all the micro-organisms – bacteria, viruses and fungi – in our gastrointestinal tract. Numerous studies have shown the enormous effect these micro-organisms have on our digestion, immune functions and overall health.[14, 15, 16, 17, 18] (Please also see 'Bowel health' on page 54.) Imbalance in these micro-organisms ('dysbiosis') can cause insulin resistance through chronic inflammation, or it can make existing insulin resistance worse. People suffering from insulin resistance have been found to have changes in their gut microbiome.

There are microbes all over our body; on our outside skin and inside skin – that is, our mucous membranes and gut lining, especially in our large intestine/bowel. There are more microbes in our bodies than there are cells with our own genetic code. There are actually only a few completely sterile areas in a healthy body, such as our blood, some areas in the nervous system and the peritoneum (the abdominal cavity that holds most of our organs). Saying that, new research evidence keeps emerging all the time as we learn more and more about the microbes in our entire body so even those 'sterile spaces' may be found not to be entirely so.

The groups of microbes we collectively call the microbiome have a function. Different types of microbes all have different roles in our body, many of them still unclear and being studied, but we do know that this microbiome actively affects many processes, including our metabolism and immune function. For example, our metabolism, energy production and absorption of nutrients all happen in co-operation with these communities of microbes. As I have said, some hormones, such as melatonin, are largely produced in the gut; the production of some other hormones elsewhere in the body is also regulated by the gut microbiome.

Chapter 2

What is called the gut–brain (or 'brain–gut') axis relates to the connection and communication between the brain and the gut. Neurons (nerve cells) in the brain, but also in our gut, are connected through the vagus nerve, with signals travelling through this nerve both ways. The brain and gut are also connected through neurotransmitters such as serotonin and GABA (gamma-aminobutyric acid), as these are produced also in the gut, as are many other chemicals which also affect the brain. All these neurotransmitters and other chemicals affect our mood and cognition. This means that an unbalanced gut microbiome does not only cause physical problems, but also mental symptoms, including depression.

Conversely, our thoughts can have a negative effect on our microbiome, affecting our immune system that way. We are all familiar with how we, for example, 'get butterflies in our stomach' when nervous, worried or scared, so it is understandable that this situation, when long term, can cause problems.

Our microbiome also communicates with our mitochondria. As discussed earlier (page 10), our metabolic health goes hand in hand with our mitochondrial health, affected by exercise, diet and our mental state. It seems that any changes in the health and balance of our gut microbiome also have direct effects on our mitochondria.

Our gut microbiome affects the health of our mitcochondria and regulates the release of many neurotransmitters and hormones

The health of our gut also affects our hormone balance. This is an important thing to remember as any problems with other hormones, such as the stress hormone cortisol, also have an effect on insulin. The microbiome regulates the release of many hormones and neurotransmitters. In addition to melatonin and serotonin, examples include GLP-1, which is a glucagon-like peptide that affects insulin and glucagon secretion, and cortisol, but also thyroid hormones and oestrogen.

When this beneficial, important gut microbiome is out of balance, it not only allows potentially pathological microbes to grow and spread, which leads to inflammation, but also affects the absorption of important micronutrients. Bacteria protect themselves by forming biofilm behind which they can safely multiply. A healthy gut microbiome forms microfilm all over bowel surfaces; without this protection the bowel lining is vulnerable.

Leaky-gut syndrome means that intestinal permeability increases, due to this inflammation. This may lead to unwanted substances, such as **microbial products** and **toxic digestive metabolites**, entering the bloodstream. This can trigger autoimmune responses, leading to chronic inflammation getting even worse which will again cause or exacerbate insulin resistance. Studies suggest that this is why people with metabolic syndrome (resulting from insulin resistance) often have some kind of inflammatory illness.[14, 15, 16, 17] Such illnesses include irritable bowel syndrome (IBS) and inflammatory bowel disease (IBD). Autoimmune illnesses, like rheumatoid arthritis, asthma, allergies and multiple sclerosis (MS), have also been thought to have some link to imbalance in the gut microbiome.

There are many things that can cause an imbalance in the microbes of the gut. For example, one single course of antibiotics can upset this balance, which can take a long time to be restored. In this situation we would only have a few types of microbe, not enough variety, and so their functions would not be what they are meant to be.

Our diet can also lead to imbalance – for example, if we don't eat enough of the vegetables that feed these beneficial bacteria. Sugary and starchy foods may also 'feed' harmful bacteria and/or yeast in the gut, leading to increased inflammation, especially if there is not enough protection from beneficial microbes.

Chapter 2

Lack of exercise

We are all aware how important regular exercise is. We are meant to move. Lack of exercise does not alone cause insulin resistance, but a sedentary lifestyle contributes to its development. Insulin plays a part in protein metabolism (please see page 5) and problems with insulin resistance will contribute to reduced muscle mass; lack of exercise would increase this tendency. And with less muscle mass there is less capacity to store glucose in the short-term (in the 'glycogen sponge' of the muscles) contributing further to pressure on sugar storage elsewhere.

Exercise is known to improve the insulin sensitivity of our cells.[18] According to many studies, even short periods of regular moderate exercise – for example, walking – have this effect,[19, 20] and this lasts for a long time after exercising. This is likely to be because physical activity helps to keep our mitochondria healthy. It increases the size and number of mitochondria, making energy production more efficient and reducing oxidative stress. Reduced numbers of mitochondria and mitochondrial dysfunction are known to be connected to insulin resistance, as discussed in Chapter 1. Lack of exercise would have an adverse effect on mitochondrial health, with reduced muscle mass. This, in addition to other lifestyle problems, can contribute to the development of insulin resistance.

Exercise improves mitochondrial health, increases muscle mass and improves our gut microbiome, all of which enhance insulin sensitivity

Regular exercise also reduces inflammation, so it is a powerful tool in preventing insulin resistance: physical activity is known to increase the amount of anti-inflammatory cytokines in the body,[19, 20] but also reduces stress hormone levels (cortisol); this in turn reduces inflammation. This could also be due to the positive effects exercise has on our gut microbiome, which seems to function better in physically active people. Exercise also increases particular hormones to help us improve our mood; one of these is serotonin. We simply feel so much better after exercising. This in turn affects our microbiome via the brain–gut axis (see page 28).

Even a small amount of regular exercise is better than no exercise at all, but, as with everything else, a good balance is important to remember. This is because over-exertion, or heavy exercise, can actually cause harm. The amount of exercise we should be doing of course depends on many things: our fitness, health, personal preference, age and body composition. We are all therefore different in what constitutes too much exercise, but we should keep in mind the importance of not causing ourselves too much stress when exercising. Excessive exercise can lead to elevated levels of cortisol, and cause hormonal imbalance in the same way other types of chronic stress can (see page 23). Our immune system could be affected as a result of over-exercising, and this could lead to increasing inflammation in the body. There is evidence that too much exercise can also damage the lining of our gut and cause leaky gut syndrome, which also leads to inflammation.[21] Again, it is difficult to say how much exercise is too much as we are all very different but, according to some experts, there are signs to look out for including: tiredness, sleep disturbance, painful muscles, poor performance, mood swings and an increased resting heart rate. Exercise is meant to make us feel good, not the opposite. Any signs of overdoing it tell us we need to rest.

Smoking and vaping

Tobacco smoking is known to decrease insulin sensitivity. Many studies have shown there is a connection between smoking and insulin resistance.[22, 23, 24, 25] One of the reason for this is likely to be that cigarette smoke contains toxins which damage mitochondria, leading to mitochondrial dysfunction, changes in their energy production and increasing levels of oxidative stress. Smokers often have reduced sensitivity to insulin, hyperinsulinaemia and changes in other metabolic markers of insulin resistance, including raised blood glucose, low HDL cholesterol and high triglyceride levels.

Smoking is also associated with elevated inflammatory markers, so mitochondrial damage as well as inflammation are thought to lie behind the development, for example, of smoking-related pulmonary diseases, such as emphysema, COPD and cancer.

In addition to interfering with insulin, smoking also affects many other hormones. The pituitary, thyroid and adrenal glands as well as testicular and ovarian functions have been found to suffer from smoking,[23] all of which problems disrupt the maintenance of a healthy hormonal balance in the body.

Smoking also affects calcium and vitamin D metabolism, increasing the risk of osteoporosis and other problems associated with lower vitamin D levels. People suffering from insulin resistance are often found to have insufficient vitamin D levels.

To avoid the harmful effects of smoking, many people have chosen to try vaping instead. E-cigarettes have become increasingly popular in recent years as a possibly healthier alternative to traditional cigarettes. However, new studies have started to emerge suggesting that vaping also increases inflammation in the lungs.[26, 27] It can cause chronic inflammation leading to problems such as asthma and COPD which would be likely to exacerbate existing insulin resistance. However, it is clear that more research is needed to understand the consequences of vaping better.

Summarising the causes of insulin resistance

To summarise this chapter, the following seem to be the most significant factors in the development of insulin resistance:
- Starch and sugar
- Advanced glycation end products (AGEs)
- Alcohol
- Refined oils, artificial trans fats and a too high ratio of omega 6 to omega 3 fatty acids
- Eating too much and too often/snacking and grazing
- Chronic stress
- Sleep disturbance
- Unbalanced gut microbiome and leaky gut syndrome[28]
- Lack of exercise
- Smoking and vaping.

Chapter 3

How do I know if I have insulin resistance?

As discussed in Chapter 2, there are many causes of insulin resistance and many problems that can make existing insulin resistance worse. What we eat every day is by far the most obvious cause for the development of its many symptoms. If our diet consists of too much carbohydrate, and especially sugar, for many years, most of us are very likely to become intolerant. In addition to excess carbohydrate, the amount of processed food on our plate today is a problem. It is not only the sugar content that causes issues, but that these foods almost always contain refined oils and trans fats, and potentially also additives which lead to inflammation, causing many symptoms and even addictions that are difficult to cope with. Processed food is often lacking vital micronutrients that we need from our diet. All this increases our risk of the many long-term consequences of insulin resistance: type 2 diabetes, stroke, heart disease, Alzheimer's disease and even cancer.

Raised insulin levels circulating in the bloodstream cause many problems in functions all over the body; all cells and tissues, including the brain, can be affected. In addition to many early signs, these metabolic and cellular problems caused by insulin resistance are believed to be behind many serious chronic illnesses and if not the sole root cause, to be a very powerful contributing factor.

Could it be Insulin Resistance?

I explained in Chapter 1 how cells in many tissues, including the liver, develop resistance to the effects of insulin. This development leads to hyperinsulinaemia, when the pancreas is secreting more and more insulin to overcome declining sensitivity to insulin. Type 2 diabetes, a well known consequence of insulin resistance, is diagnosed when this cycle keeps going – probably for many years – with increasing amounts of insulin in the body and worsening resistance to it, until eventually blood sugar levels stay above the normal range.

By this time, the situation has developed to a stage where blood glucose levels can no longer be controlled by the body's compensating mechanism. Instead, this mechanism starts to fail. It is likely that insulin resistance has been present for many years before this happens, causing many other problems in the body during that time. As discussed previously, we are all very different in the way our body reacts to problems with insulin; we all have a different genetic makeup. For some of us, insulin resistance eventually leads to heart disease, whereas others are diagnosed with an autoimmune disease. Some of us put on weight at a very young age, while for others excess weight is not a big problem. However, too much insulin in the body causes serious problems for all of us eventually.

Too much insulin in the body causes different health issues depending on our genetic makeup but in the end it causes serious problems for all of us

I don't think most of us have actually understood how deeply this problem affects the whole body. We have not realised how many increasingly common symptoms there are with no obvious known cause, such as fatigue, aches and pains or depression, which are most likely caused by insulin resistance. Insulin resistance is a far more serious problem than we ever thought before, but unfortunately it is still rarely discussed in connection with conditions other than type 2 diabetes. However, the link is obvious, both in the scientific literature and also in practice.

It is difficult sometimes to know for sure if we suffer from insulin resistance because fasting insulin levels, which would be a good marker of insulin resistance, are not usually tested in primary care. However; even without any tests, there are many signs and symptoms that are very likely caused by insulin resistance. The more of these signs there are, the worse insulin resistance is likely to be. Remember that diabetes is only one of the complications of insulin resistance. Most people with the problem have a completely normal blood glucose level, only raised insulin levels. Measuring the blood glucose level is therefore not a reliable indicator of insulin resistance.

The most common signs and symptoms of insulin resistance are:
- excess weight
- low blood sugar levels (hypoglycaemia) which cause crashing between meals
- constant tiredness and low energy levels
- mood swings
- snoring and sleep apnoea
- many skin problems, including skin tags
- recurring inner ear problems
- raised blood pressure
- raised triglyceride and low HDL levels in our cholesterol check.

Insulin has many functions in the body, as we have seen (see Table 1 on page 4), including but not confined to managing glucose metabolism, and these many symptoms stem from this range.

Expanding waistline, weight gain and obesity

Weight gain is usually a very good sign of insulin resistance. In fact, it can be the only sign. If we are overweight, and especially if there is excess weight in the abdomen, it is very likely that we suffer from insulin resistance. Not all people with this condition are overweight but they are likely to have more weight than they should have around their midriff. Our waist to height ratio is a good way of assessing insulin resistance. It is done by measuring the waist and comparing the result with our height. If our waist measurement is more than half of our height measurement, we are likely to be suffering from insulin resistance.

We will discuss obesity in more detail later in this book (page 47).

Hypoglycaemia – *low* blood sugar levels

One of the symptoms of insulin resistance is a condition called 'hypoglycaemia' – low blood sugar levels. If there are high levels of insulin in the body, as a result of eating a lot of carbohydrates and especially sugar, it is likely that between meals the blood sugar levels will come crashing down, often below normal. Low blood sugar makes us feel tired, low and irritable and causes 'brain fog', which makes it difficult to concentrate.

We associate type 2 diabetes with hyperglycaemia (too high blood sugar), but in insulin resistance blood sugar comes crashing down between meals and can wake us in the night

Many people also experience problems with their working memory. This is most likely caused by low energy levels as there is not enough glucose in the brain, or there are problems with glucose metabolism, which leads to reduced cognitive function. We will discuss the effects of insulin resistance on our brain in Chapter 4 (see page 66).

Hypoglycaemia also causes food cravings which are often very difficult to control. We might also constantly feel hungry and need snacks, crave carbohydrates and especially sugar and, as a result, eat too much and too often. Many of us tend to try to fix these problems with eating many snacks during the day, which will only make the situation worse in the long run. We are not meant to eat too often, as I have said.

Hypoglycaemia puts our body into panic mode – we release adrenaline to get our blood sugar level back up to normal. This might make us feel hot, shaky and anxious and even wake us up at night.

Tiredness, low energy levels and mood swings

As described earlier, fluctuating blood sugar levels can cause regular tiredness, lethargy and mood swings. Many people with unstable blood sugar levels feel they have very little energy and are tired even when sleeping reasonably well. As a result of insulin resistance, fuel in the form of sugar cannot enter the cells when needed so the cells cannot make the energy (ATP) they need; alternatively, mitochondrial dysfunction caused by insulin resistance may affect energy production. Our mood might also be affected by the hormonal imbalance caused by insulin resistance. All these factors together can be detrimental to our mental health.

Low immunity

We have already discussed inflammation and the link between chronic inflammation and insulin resistance. It seems that many people suffering from insulin resistance and related conditions and problems, also suffer from recurrent acute infections, such as common colds, coughs and flu-like illnesses, as well as skin infections, as discussed below. One 'meta-analysis' (systematic review) of all published research found that people with diabetes were also more prone to post-surgery infections,[1] so the risk of all types of infection is likely to be higher in people with insulin resistance even when they have not (yet) developed diabetes. Many of my patients suffering from metabolic problems find that it is difficult for them to fight off even cold-like infections and they are more likely to get complications, such as bacterial chest infections.

One study has found that insulin boosts the functioning of a type of immune cell called a T-cell during immune responses to fighting infections, such as the flu virus.[2] Insulin resistance interfered with this function, because the cells can't respond to insulin as they should. The body's immune system as a whole does not then function properly as a result.

I am writing this book during the worldwide coronavirus pandemic of 2019 (Covid-19). It is becoming more and more obvious that metabolic problems caused by insulin resistance, as well as associated inflammation, are factors that increase the risks of complications of this disease. Studies in this area are still ongoing and the exact reason for this is currently unclear. When an association between insulin resistance and Covid-19 is confirmed, more effort should be put towards treating underlying insulin resistance in order to prevent complications.

Another cause of low immunity is likely to be an unbalanced gut microbiome, often linked to insulin resistance as I explained earlier (see page 26). Chronic inflammation might also have an effect if our body is already 'battling' against ongoing inflammation with not enough energy available for our immune responses to fight off an acute infection. The risk of acute infection is also higher if there is a chronic inflammatory condition in the background that is being treated with medication, such as steroids, that affects immunity.

We will talk about the liver in more detail in Chapter 4, but it is important to point out here that it has a big role in our immune response. Since we know insulin resistance is involved in the development of fatty liver disease, it is likely that the immune functions of the liver are affected as a result of such damage to this organ.

Snoring and sleep apnoea

Sleep apnoea is a serious condition in which there are breaks in breathing during sleep. Usually gasping or snorting noises can be heard during these breaks as well as heavy snoring. Sleep is constantly disturbed, which leads to increased tiredness during the day.

Sleep apnoea is closely linked to chronic conditions such as obesity and high blood pressure; it is also one of the common signs of insulin resistance. It causes stress in the body due to low oxygen, inflammation increasing even further, making insulin resistance worse.

Even without sleep apnoea, snoring can affect our lives. It causes sleep disruption, which may lead to chronic stress. This problem too has been linked to metabolic issues through chronic inflammation and obesity. Many of my patients have told me that snoring has significantly reduced very quickly after taking measures to reverse their insulin resistance.

Skin problems, including skin tags

There are many common skin conditions linked to insulin resistance. One of them is increased numbers of skin tags. This connection has been found in many studies, but the exact mechanism is unknown. However, it is thought that insulin as a growth-stimulating hormone is behind this as hyperinsulinaemia causes alterations in the normal levels of insulin-like growth factor (IGF) and also affects normal functioning of growth hormone.

A condition called **acanthosis nigricans** is also linked to insulin resistance. This is where areas of darker discolouration develop on the skin, usually in the armpits, neck or groin. This is caused by rapid reproduction of epidermal (outer layer) cells in the skin, thought to be due to raised levels of insulin, because of its growth-stimulating effect.

Insulin resistance is also linked to many inflammatory skin conditions, such as acne and hidradenitis suppurativa. The latter is a condition which causes painful cyst-like lumps and boils on the skin, many of them inflamed, leaking pus and leading to scarring of the skin. Mostly these lumps develop in the armpits, groin and below the breasts, but they can occur in other parts of the body. These problems are thought to be linked to the hormonal imbalance caused by insulin resistance, but also to related inflammation.

People suffering from diabetes are known to be more prone to many infections, both bacterial – such as cellulitis (an infection of one of the layers of the skin) – and fungal infections, such as thrush, athletes' foot or 'jock itch'. Reduced immune function associated with chronic inflammation and insulin resistance, discussed earlier (page 37), is likely to be one of the reasons for an overgrowth of microbes such as yeast or disease-causing ('pathogenic') bacteria.

Inner ear problems, including tinnitus

Inner ear problems, such as dizziness, vertigo and/or tinnitus, have been found to be connected to problems with carbohydrate metabolism and insulin resistance. This is thought to be because the structures in the inner ear become dysfunctional as a result of associated poor glucose delivery into the cells. Just as with many other tissues, metabolism in the inner ear is very active and so any changes in the metabolic balance in the body affect the area.

There are always many other possible causes for ear/hearing

conditions, but metabolic problems should always be kept in mind when trying to treat recurring inner ear problems.

Raised blood pressure

Although there are a few other causes for raised blood pressure, the most common is metabolic syndrome resulting from insulin resistance. Insulin causes salt to accumulate in the kidneys and the body generally, which leads in turn to raised blood pressure. Very often people with elevated blood pressure readings also have other signs of insulin resistance, such as excess weight.

Higher than normal blood pressure readings are a good marker for insulin resistance. Even with reasonably good blood pressure, people suffering from insulin resistance often also have problems with swelling, especially in their feet and ankles, because of fluid retention. High insulin levels, and the inflammation they cause, can also thicken the smooth muscle around blood vessels, which contributes to high blood pressure.

When insulin resistance is treated, raised blood pressure returns to normal levels for most people, usually very quickly.

A normal blood pressure reading is around 120/80 mm Hg. The first reading, 120 here, is called 'systolic blood pressure' and the other, 80, 'diastolic blood pressure'. If the blood pressure reading is 140/90 or above, it is considered to be raised. It is normal, however, for the systolic blood pressure reading to be higher when we get older, because of the natural changes in our blood vessels. Therefore, the limit for normal blood pressure is 150/90 for people aged 80 and over (NHS England).[3]

It is important to maintain a normal blood pressure as, if the pressure is too high, it can damage the blood vessels and increase the risk of heart disease and stroke. We are often told only to avoid salt in order to manage our blood pressure. When our blood pressure is high and/or we suffer from swelling in our legs, it is advisable to reduce the amount of salt, but salt is not usually the root cause – insulin is. If insulin resistance is treated, blood pressure almost always returns to normal and swelling reduces.

Cholesterol: low HDL cholesterol and high triglyceride levels

Cholesterol is an important substance in all our cells. It is the main structural component of cells and therefore of all tissues in the body. It is also needed in hormone synthesis, cell regeneration and absorption of fat-soluble vitamins, and so is an absolutely necessary substance for life. Our body makes most of the cholesterol it needs, mainly in the liver, but we also receive it from our diet, from foods such as organ meat, eggs and shellfish. Because of our own cholesterol production, it does not make much difference if we get cholesterol from our diet or not – if we eat more cholesterol-rich foods, our liver produces less cholesterol and vice versa.

When our cholesterol levels are measured by our doctor, we usually get a result for total cholesterol levels and also for its components: HDL, LDL and triglycerides. There are different opinions on what these readings should be. NHS England currently recommends:

total cholesterol: 5 or below

HDL: above 1

LDL: 3 or below

triglycerides: below 2.

The NHS refers to HDL as 'good cholesterol' and LDL as 'bad cholesterol', and many of us know that we should not have too much 'bad' cholesterol in our bloodstream. However, the cholesterol issue is much more complex than this. It seems that instead of looking at the overall total cholesterol or LDL cholesterol, we should concentrate particularly on HDL cholesterol and triglycerides. This is because low levels of HDL and high levels of triglycerides are associated with insulin resistance and therefore the most important feature when looking at metabolic syndrome. This is a harmful combination.

Going back to Chapter 1 where I discussed our metabolism, I explained that fatty acids, as well as the cholesterol we eat and the cholesterol our liver produces, are largely made up of triglycerides and transported through the bloodstream in lipoproteins. There are two different lipoproteins – low density lipoprotein (LDL) and high density lipoprotein (HDL). The cholesterol values for LDL and HDL measure how much cholesterol is carried in these lipoprotein particles in the bloodstream. LDL is still often referred as 'bad' cholesterol because high LDL levels have previously been thought to be linked to an increased risk of heart disease. So it is very likely to be an important part of the cholesterol profile to determine our metabolic health. However, many studies have found that we should not look at the overall amount of LDL as such, as not all LDL is the same. It is the size of those LDL particles that matters.

There is not just one type of LDL cholesterol, but two: type A (large dense LDL) and type B (small dense LDL). It is the latter that is considered to be the dangerous type, and most likely to be associated with heart disease. These small LDL particles can enter the artery wall and become oxidised causing inflammation. The size of LDL particles is determined by how much sugar is in our diet. The carbohydrates we eat, which are essentially sugar as we have seen, damage the LDL particles in our blood, changing them to these smaller particles.

Not all LDL cholesterol is bad – it is the size of the particles that matters and their size is determined by the amount of sugar we eat

HDL is referred to as 'good cholesterol', as already mentioned, because it brings cholesterol back to the liver from the rest of the body to be processed and eliminated.

Triglyceride levels in the blood also rise when the dietary carbohydrate intake is high. They are made by the liver, from excess carbohydrates, and transported in lipoproteins in the bloodstream. Raised triglyceride levels are associated with heart disease and insulin resistance; very high levels are dangerous because they can cause inflammation of the pancreas (pancreatitis).

The HDL-to-triglyceride ratio is actually a very good way of measuring insulin resistance. Often when insulin resistance is present, HDL cholesterol may be low, but triglycerides will certainly be raised.

It is good to remember that cholesterol in itself is not something we have to worry about too much, in contrast to what we were taught in the past. High levels do not necessarily mean unhealthy levels. When insulin resistance is treated properly, HDL levels usually go up and triglyceride levels come down. LDL levels might increase, but this is most likely to be the large-molecule, more harmless LDL. Also, chronic inflammation goes down when insulin resistance is treated, which is much more important – chronic inflammation is, as we have seen, the initial cause of the development of chronic illnesses such as heart disease.

Summarising the signs and symptoms of insulin resistance

In summary, signs that you may have insulin resistance include:
- fat around the middle with a low waist-to-height ratio
- crashing between meals
- being tired all the time
- having low/irritable mood, brain fog and/or mood swings

Chapter 3

- food cravings and/or constant snacking
- recurrent infections
- snoring and/or sleep apnoea
- skin problems: tags, acne, hidradenitis suppurativa, dark patches (acanthus nigricans)
- tinnitus, dizziness and/or vertigo
- swollen feet and ankles
- raised blood pressure
- high triglyceride levels.

Chapter 4

What are the consequences of insulin resistance?

Excess weight

Most people battling with excess weight know already that it is a question of much more than just calories. Most obese people have tried numerous diets to lose weight, but have found it an impossible task. Often losing weight has only been possible through eating less, but the wrong foods, so that the dieter is hungry and battles with constant cravings. Losing weight this way often results in gaining even more once the diet is over. This is probably because our weight is hormonally regulated and just by eating less it is difficult to change our hormones. Obesity is mainly caused by insulin resistance and having too much insulin in the body, rather than eating too many calories.

Our weight is hormonally regulated and it is difficult to change our hormones just by eating less

As we have seen, insulin is responsible for the storage of glucose as fat in our bodies and this is how we gain weight. Insulin also prevents the burning of this stored fat, so if we have too much insulin in our body all the time because of insulin resistance, there is no fat burning – only storage. It becomes almost impossible in these circumstances to lose weight. High insulin levels mean that the opposite hormone to insulin –

glucagon – is always low, which means the body cannot use stored energy; it cannot burn the fat. To do that, we need to lower levels of insulin, rather than reduce calories.

Children and young people in particular are at risk of putting on weight as a result of problems with insulin. They are very sensitive to hormonal imbalances and statistics show that more and more children are overweight. With a better understanding of the part insulin plays, we have a better chance of helping young people and reversing the obesity epidemic. Poor diet not only affects this generation, but also the next when babies born from mothers suffering from insulin resistance are already relatively large when born, and have an increased risk of becoming obese later in life; often this is already manifest in childhood.

To burn stored energy (fat) we need to lower insulin levels rather than calories

It seems that existing maternal insulin resistance during pregnancy has many affects in the placenta, adversely affecting its proper functioning which can lead to problems with transportation of nutrients to the unborn baby. There is a greater risk of gestational diabetes and studies done within this area show that an increased risk of metabolic disease for the baby later in life is not only caused by inherited eating habits, but also by epigenetic changes caused by exposure to maternal diabetes.[1, 2] We will talk more about insulin resistance in pregnancy in Chapter 6 (page 112).

Fatty liver

The liver is an essential organ that is central to our metabolic functioning. We cannot survive without the liver. It processes, stores and releases nutrients and eliminates wastes.

Chapter 4

The liver helps to break down fat in our diet and stores or releases it as energy. It also stores extra glucose as glycogen, breaks down proteins and metabolises fructose (fruit sugar discussed before – page 17), alcohol and any medication we have taken. The liver also has a big role in our immune system.

Its role in glucose metabolism involves not only storing glucose but also producing it according to our body's needs. This process, as mentioned earlier, is called 'gluconeogenesis' and this is regulated by insulin so that when we eat and have enough glucose in the body from our food, the liver's production stops.

The liver also converts excess carbohydrates into fat (triglycerides).

Non-alcoholic fatty liver disease (NAFLD) has recently become a very common diagnosis (see page 17). 'Fatty liver' means that there is a buildup of fat in the liver cells. Normally there is only very little, or no fat in the liver, but in the development of this condition, abnormal amounts start to accumulate there. Insulin resistance eventually affects all organs in the body, including the liver. Chronic inflammation, caused by excess fat in the liver, increases the risk of insulin resistance in this organ. When the liver develops insulin resistance, it continues producing glucose even when insulin is present and there is already enough glucose. This will speed up insulin resistance, making it worse elsewhere in the body also and in this way contribute to the development of type 2 diabetes. (We will discuss diabetes in more detail later – see page 59.)

In summary, the chain of events is like this:[3, 4]

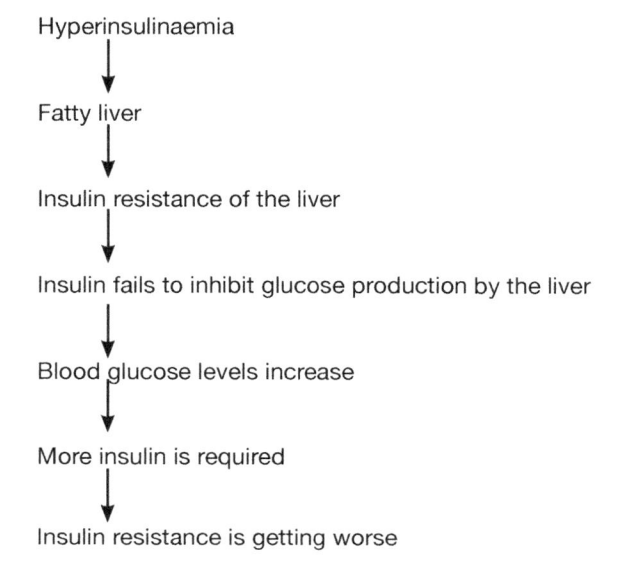

Hyperinsulinaemia
↓
Fatty liver
↓
Insulin resistance of the liver
↓
Insulin fails to inhibit glucose production by the liver
↓
Blood glucose levels increase
↓
More insulin is required
↓
Insulin resistance is getting worse

In addition to glucose production, in the presence of insulin resistance the liver increases its production of fat to store the glucose, which results in increasing amounts of triglycerides also in the bloodstream. This will increase our risk of, for example, heart disease.

The reason for NAFLD's development is excess carbohydrate, especially fructose which is converted into liver fat as explained previously. Negative changes in the gut microbiome may also contribute to the development of fatty liver due to inflammation.

Fatty liver can be a serious condition. There are usually no symptoms at an early stage, with the only sign being weight gain in our midriff. This is, however, a good sign of insulin resistance that needs our attention. This is because, in many cases, the condition can lead to the development of a more serious liver problem – fibrosis, where inflammation caused by the fat accumulation starts to cause permanent scarring, a situation which can lead to cirrhosis and even liver cancer.

In addition to the liver, extra fat often starts to accumulate in other organs too. Fatty pancreas is likewise a problem, increasing inflammation and insulin resistance throughout the body in its turn. Like fatty liver, it can be serious as it has been closely associated with pancreatic cancer.

Hormone imbalance including polycystic ovary syndrome (PCOS)

Many hormonal problems are linked to insulin resistance. These problems include early puberty, thyroid problems and polycystic ovary syndrome (PCOS). Insulin is a hormone (chemical messenger) and, as explained previously (page 5), any problems with one hormone in our finely balanced hormone system will cause problems in other hormones too. In other words, insulin resistance affects our overall hormone (endocrine) system.

PCOS is an example of such a complication. Too much insulin affects the ovaries and causes them to overproduce testosterone. This prevents normal ovulation and can lead to infertility. PCOS also causes many other, often very distressing symptoms, such as acne, hair loss, facial hair, obesity and irregular and/or heavy periods. Treating insulin resistance with a low-carb diet (see Chapter 7) always helps the body return to its normal hormonal balance and this helps relieve symptoms of conditions like PCOS.

Endometriosis, another very distressing problem, associated with episodic severe pelvic pain, is a condition where tissue that women normally have lining their womb (uterus) – the endometrium – grows in areas of the pelvis outside of the womb or the fallopian tubes. This causes pelvic pain and problems with heavy periods and pain during periods. The cause of endometriosis in unclear, but many patients who suffer from endometriosis also suffer from PCOS, suggesting a link with insulin resistance. Also, the symptoms are often similar in both of these conditions, and in addition to other problems, endometriosis has been thought to be associated with hormonal imbalance and problems with the immune system, both of which are present in other conditions linked to insulin resistance. Endometriosis has also been found to have links with many autoimmune conditions. Finally, it is often misdiagnosed as IBS (see page 54) and the two conditions often co-occur.

'Oestrogen dominance' is a condition where there are high levels of oestrogen in the body compared with progesterone levels. There are many symptoms of this imbalance, including tiredness, problems with periods (heavy, painful, irregular etc), mood swings, hair loss, weight gain, sleep problems and bloating. Again, the knock-on effect of insulin dysregulation can be this imbalance between oetrogen and progesterone.

Thyroid hormones have an important role in glucose metabolism and often people who suffer from problems with thyroid function also have insulin resistance. Insulin has been shown to interfere with the functioning of the thyroid gland[5, 6, 7] which causes abnormalities in the production of thyroid hormones and how cells respond to them.

Meanwhile, several adrenal disorders, with increased secretion of adrenocortical hormones, are also linked to insulin resistance. These include Cushing's syndrome, which is a condition where too much cortisol is secreted in the body, and Addison's disease, when the adrenal glands eventually fail.

In men, a condition called **benign prostate enlargement**, which is very common in older men, is also linked to insulin resistance. Insulin causes the growth of the prostate (remember, it is a growth promoter – see page 5), but changes in sex hormones as well as inflammation are also thought to contribute. Insulin resistance is also linked to prostate cancer.

Gynaecomastia – enlarged breast tissue in men ('man boobs') – with or without significant obesity, is caused by hormonal imbalances related to insulin resistance, usually higher than normal oestrogen levels.

Insulin resistance should be considered with any condition involving a hormone imbalance

Insulin resistance should be considered when treating any of these conditions. In addition to metabolic problems, the overall hormonal balance is likely to be affected if there are problems with the microbiome balance in the gut. As discussed in Chapter 2, the gut microbes affect the production of many hormones in our body.

Mouth and dental problems

Inflammation in the mouth and gums is another complication of insulin resistance. Dental conditions such as periodontitis (inflammation of the supporting structures of the teeth), gum disease and also tooth decay (dental caries) are all linked not only with diabetes but also with insulin resistance.

The reasons for these problems are the same as for all other parts of the body affected by insulin resistance – persistent metabolic disturbance, high dietary carbohydrate intake, decreased intake/absorption of micronutrients, chronic inflammation and immune dysfunction. More specifically, the microbiome in the mouth has a big part to play. If its balance is disturbed, the situation gives way to the growth of harmful bacteria and fungi, increasing the risk of infection and tooth decay. Poor oral hygiene contributes to the development of these conditions as well as the use of antibacterial or antiseptic mouthwashes. These mouthwashes may harm the oral microbiome, the 'good' bacteria in the mouth which protect against harmful bacteria. Without this natural protection we are more prone to tooth decay.

Osteoporosis

It seems that insulin resistance affects bone health just as it does dental, causing a reduction in bone density. Worryingly, this is being found not only in older people but in young adults too. Bone is a metabolically active organ, just like many other tissues, and can suffer from inflammation associated with insulin resistance as well as a lack of nutrients, which leads to mitochondrial dysfunction. The link between osteoporosis and mitochondrial dysfunction is well recognised. If our mitochondria are not functioning properly (see Chapter 1), the normal processes in the bones are disrupted. These involve two types of bone cells – osteoblasts that build bone tissue and osteoclasts that break it down in a constant process of renewal and repair.

Bowel problems

The gut microbiome and its connection with healthy functioning of the body was discussed in Chapter 2. Problems that arise when the microbiome is out of balance include leaky gut syndrome and chronic inflammation, which lead to insulin resistance, as well as many other chronic conditions, as discussed already.

This chain of events largely explains why people with insulin resistance and metabolic syndrome usually also have bowel problems of one sort or another. These problems include irritable bowel syndrome (IBS) and the more severe inflammatory bowel diseases (IBD).

IBS affects the colon mainly, but also other parts of the digestive system, causing symptoms such as abdominal cramping, bloating, constipation and diarrhoea. It is very likely to have a link with insulin resistance – many people who suffer from insulin resistance also have IBS-type symptoms.[8, 9] This may well relate to diet. High consumption of carbohydrates, especially refined sugar and flour, often leads to other abdominal symptoms, with common complaints being constipation and acid reflux.

IBD, which includes ulcerative colitis and Crohn's disease, is more severe, with abdominal cramps and swelling, but also pain, bloody diarrhoea, tiredness and weight loss in many patients. Inflammation can become so severe that sections of the bowel have to be removed and there is also an increased risk of colon cancer with IBD. IBD has been linked with dysbiosis (unbalanced gut microbiome) and inflammation associated with insulin resistance but also with an original infection. Its development is very complex. However, in treating this condition, the focus should be on both inflammation and the microbiome. I have seen many people manage the symptoms very well when insulin resistance was treated and measures to reduce inflammation implemented (please read more about dietary measures in Chapter 5). This would be an extremely important approach to avoid difficult and life-changing medical treatments, such as immuno-suppressants and even surgery.

Insulin resistance can also cause a condition called **autonomic neuropathy (AN)**, common especially in diabetic patients. Constipation is a very common symptom in this condition which involves damage to the nerves controlling involuntary functions in the body. When the condition affects the vagus nerve, gastroparesis can develop. Gastroparesis causes problems with digestion and emptying of the stomach, leading to symptoms such as bloating and heartburn (oesophageal reflux). In addition to stomach and bowel functions, this condition can affect many other organs, causing symptoms all over the body. These symptoms include dizziness, night sweats and problems with bladder functions. Sometimes, for example, frequent urinary tract infections or urinary incontinence are caused by AN.

It is difficult to diagnose AN as many symptoms are similar to symptoms caused by other conditions. Treatment is symptomatic but again should always include measures to reduce insulin resistance and restore the hormonal and metabolic balance in the body.

Chronic pain

By 'chronic' pain we mean pain that lasts for several weeks, or even months or years. It can affect any part of our body and often occurs for no apparent reason – no injury or acute infection. Alternatively, it may start with an injury, such as a pulled muscle, but does not get better, or keeps recurring. There are also specific health conditions associated with chronic pain, the most common being fibromyalgia, chronic fatigue syndrome and endometriosis. Inflammatory bowel disease also causes ongoing abdominal pain, as discussed earlier.

Fibromyalgia is a complicated condition with symptoms of pain all over the body, tiredness and often mental health problems, such as depression, poor memory and inability to concentrate. Many patients also suffer from abdominal symptoms similar to irritable bowel syndrome (IBS). Recent study has indeed suggested a link to insulin resistance,[10] something that many clinicians had already been thinking about for a long time. It makes sense since fibromyalgia often goes hand in hand with other conditions associated with insulin resistance, such as endometriosis, hypothyroidism and other autoimmune diseases.[11] In my practice, I have found that the symptoms of many patients improve significantly when insulin resistance is treated in the right way. (We will discuss reversing insulin resistance in the next chapter.) The exact mechanism by which insulin resistance causes the symptoms is not clear, but they are thought to be connected with chronic inflammation and reduced mitochondrial activity. Alterations in the central nervous system with pain signaling and in the immune system have also been found in patients suffering from fibromyalgia, which connects the condition to having an unbalanced microbiome. A study published in 2019 supported this possibility.[12]

The gut microbiome acts as a modulator of many types of

pain, including inflammatory pain, neuropathic pain and headache, through the gut–brain axis.

Chronic fatigue syndrome (CFS) is another complicated condition, severely affecting the lives of many patients. It is also known by many other names, including myalgic encephalomyelitis (ME). Symptoms are very similar to fibromyalgia, and include extreme tiredness, pain and sleep disturbances. Often the symptoms are worse after physical exertion which affects the patients' ability to handle their usual daily activities. Resting does not seem to help them. Many might also experience cognitive problems, such as poor concentration and memory. While the cause of CFS is still officially unknown, it has been associated with the same problems we see in insulin resistance – low immunity and hormone imbalances. Just as with fibromyalgia, insulin resistance is a likely root cause of CFS also.

Chronic pain, wherever it is experienced, as well as continuing fatigue, are very difficult for the patient. These are all debilitating conditions, often leading to depression. Because the underlying conditions discussed are so difficult to diagnose and often no known cause for the symptoms can be found, many patients feel that they are not being taken seriously. It is particularly important to try to find the root cause of chronic pain and, whatever the situation, it is always worth trying lifestyle interventions, as in Chapter 5, to reverse insulin resistance. It usually has a very beneficial effect.

Peripheral neuropathy

Peripheral neuropathy is a condition affecting the peripheral nervous system in which the nerves in the extremities – the hands and feet mainly – are damaged. Symptoms include pain, weakness and tingling or loss of sensation. Peripheral neuropathy is usually linked to diabetes, but it seems that elevated insulin levels alone can cause it even when blood sugar levels are within normal limits.[13, 14] It could be that it is insulin that is the root cause in this condition also, rather than high blood glucose. Peripheral neuropathy can lead to serious complications, such as foot ulcers and even gangrene if infection is present, leading eventually to foot/limb amputation.

It is important to be aware that vitamin B_{12} deficiency can also cause neuropathy. Vitamin B_{12} is an essential vitamin which we get from animal-based foods, such as meat and eggs, and/or from supplements, especially when there are no animal-based foods in our diet. Abdominal problems, such as imbalance in the gut microbiome, might affect the absorption of this important vitamin, so if we experience any symptoms of B_{12} deficiency, it is important to discuss these with a doctor.

Absorption of vitamin B_{12} can also be compromised by many prescribed drugs, including the diabetes drug metformin and proton pump inhibitors, such as omeprazole, and by conditions such as IBD that damage the gut lining, and by ileostomy (removal of the last section of the small bowel). People with pernicious anaemia cannot absorb B_{12} at all from their food and need regular injections of the vitamin for life.

Gout

There is a strong link between gout, obesity and metabolic syndrome, so insulin resistance is again likely to be the root cause. Gout occurs where there are elevated uric acid levels in the body, resulting in crystals being deposited in the affected joint(s), usually the base of the great toe. This causes inflammation, swelling and severe pain. Patients suffering from gout are often told to avoid meat. This is because uric acid is a breakdown product of purines, a building block of the proteins that meat contains. It used to be thought therefore that gout was caused by eating too much red meat in particular. However, it has been found that having high levels of insulin increases uric acid levels and causes gout symptoms.[15] This is thought to be because of decreasing excretion of uric acid by the kidneys.

Fructose (fruit sugar) and alcohol also both increase uric acid levels in the blood. When the body breaks down fructose and/or alcohol, purines are released. Again, treating insulin resistance has been effective in treating gout too.

Type 2 diabetes

Type 2 diabetes is a known complication of insulin resistance. It is diagnosed when blood sugar levels are constantly elevated. It is very important to note that type 2 diabetes is not a problem with high blood sugar levels as such, but is a metabolic problem with the hormone insulin. However, as discussed earlier, type 2 diabetes is a late finding of insulin resistance, developing at an advanced stage. Insulin resistance often starts many years before blood sugar levels begin to be above normal. The damage insulin resistance causes often goes unnoticed for long periods if we concentrate only on blood sugar levels rather than other signs of insulin resistance. This is a huge problem because, compared with the number of type 2 diabetics, the number of people with insulin resistance is likely to be much, much higher. If we focused more on insulin resistance, we could recognise it better and reverse it long before diabetes set in.

With insulin resistance, over time the body's ability to compensate starts to fail. Even though more insulin is being pumped into the bloodstream to try and control all that glucose, when the cells have developed resistance, that resistance only keeps getting worse, and more and more glucose eventually stays in the bloodstream. The glucose is unable to enter the cells and so blood glucose levels keep getting higher. First, they are only just above normal levels, in a condition called 'pre-diabetes'. If no lifestyle changes are made, the situation is progressive and full-blown type 2 diabetes will be just around the corner.

As discussed previously, insulin resistance affects all organs in the body, including the liver. When the liver develops insulin resistance, it will make insulin resistance worse elsewhere and possibly lead to type 2 diabetes more quickly. Insulin resistance in the liver results in worsening uncontrolled sugar production there, which causes raised blood sugar levels even in the mornings after the nightly fast. This so-called 'dawn phenomenon' is normal, with many other hormones promoting this glucose production, including glucagon and cortisol, to stop our blood sugar levels from dropping too low over night when we are not eating and also giving us energy for the day ahead. In healthy people, insulin regulates this well, but if the liver's sensitivity to insulin is reduced, blood sugar levels continue to rise depending on how severe the insulin resistance is. Many people suffering from type 2 diabetes notice this as raised blood glucose levels in the mornings.

Type 2 diabetes is not to be taken lightly. I know that many of my patients, for example, do not realise how dangerous this disease is as, in the beginning, there may not be many clear symptoms at all and the diagnosis often comes as a surprise. I think that some people are not too concerned also because of the fact that this has become so common. 'Everyone', especially in a certain age group, has diabetes. However, the diagnosis should be taken very seriously. Without proper changes in lifestyle this is a progressive disease that will lead to difficult complications such as kidney failure, blindness and/or amputations as the extensive damage caused by raised insulin levels, together with elevated blood sugar levels, affects the whole body and all its tissues, all the time.

There are a number of medications available for controlling blood sugar levels, including metformin mentioned above in relation to vitamin B_{12} deficiency. However, medication does not treat the cause of diabetes, only the symptoms. Without lifestyle measures it is impossible to reverse this disease and it is progressive. When we understand the problem with too much insulin in the body and insulin resistance, we also understand

Chapter 4

that the only way of treating type 2 diabetes is to reduce the amount of insulin in the body, which means reducing the amount of carbohydrate and cutting out sugar especially from our diet. If we continue to eat a diet high in carbohydrates, and rely only on medication to control our high blood sugar, the root problem with insulin resistance will only continue to get worse. It will become more and more difficult to control blood sugar levels with medication.

Using insulin to treat this illness is simply the wrong approach. Injecting even more insulin into the body in this situation is very harmful. It will help to control blood sugar levels for a while, but it will add further to the problem of hyperinsulinaemia and its effects, making insulin resistance much worse. Patients using insulin will nearly always go on to develop complications. I can understand that insulin treatment might be the only option in patients unable or unwilling to make any changes to their diet; those extremely high blood sugar levels need to be controlled somehow. However, too many patients don't understand the problem with insulin and might see insulin treatment as an easy option. It is not. Lifestyle changes are absolutely necessary to avoid complications.

Although type 2 diabetes is chronic and progressive, this is only actually true if the diet remains the same. If people with the condition reduce their intake of sugar and other carbohydrates that caused the disease in the first place, they can usually reduce or even stop their diabetes medications. This is common sense. Having diabetes means that you are carbohydrate-intolerant and you cannot go on eating carbohydrate in the way you used to. We need to understand this and then we will be fine. Type 2 diabetes can be reversed. Treating diabetes with a diet low in carbohydrates is extremely effective. If we add intermittent fasting to the diet, this treatment is particularly powerful. Blood glucose and HbA1C (see page 19) levels return and stay within normal levels for most patients.

Important note: Please remember that if you are taking insulin or another medication for your type 2 diabetes, you will need to be careful when starting a diet low in carbohydrates. Your blood sugar levels will start to settle quickly, so taking insulin or some other medications might be dangerous. Please see your doctor before starting a low-carbohydrate diet and you will have to monitor your own blood sugar levels carefully.

Heart disease

Coronary heart disease affects the blood vessels supplying the heart with blood. The main symptoms are angina (heart pain), heart attacks and heart failure. Lifestyle and diet are known to be the biggest drivers of heart disease. This means that we can do a lot ourselves to prevent it.

However, there has been a lot of confusion in recent years about nutrition and heart disease, especially around natural saturated fat. In the past we have been told to avoid fat altogether, for our heart health. There are a growing number of scientists and doctors at the moment, however, who very strongly believe that natural fats and/or cholesterol do not cause heart disease but, just the opposite, help to avoid it. Looking at the science, there is no proof that natural saturated fat, such as butter, is dangerous; on the contrary, heart disease is thought to be a part of the many other problems caused mostly by low-grade inflammation and insulin resistance, together with lack of exercise, stress and smoking. Vascular inflammation caused by these factors damages the artery walls, which leads to atherosclerosis and heart disease.

I explained LDL cholesterol earlier (page 43), and how it is the size of LDL particles that matters rather than the number. Also that HDL cholesterol and triglyceride levels matter, not the total amount of cholesterol. An unhealthy cholesterol profile is linked to insulin resistance, not dietary fat intake. Sugar and insulin damage the arterial walls, as mentioned previously, and for this reason it is known that fluctuating sugar levels are especially harmful. Cholesterol, among other substances, forms a patch to cover the damage, so we know cholesterol is present in these situations, but it is not the initial cause of the damage.

We don't know exactly what cholesterol's role is in the development of heart disease, especially when there is a family history of very high cholesterol levels – hypercholesterolaemia – but it seems very clear that we have exaggerated its role in the past while we have ignored the role of sugar and insulin resistance more or less completely. Having feared fat for decades, believing that saturated fat causes heart disease despite science showing the opposite, it will take a long time for ideas about saturated fat to change.

On the other hand, as already mentioned, increasing numbers of healthcare professionals are aware of the problems associated with insulin resistance and, like me, are keen to find out more about it, to be able to help their patients. Many of the old guidelines are also changing. British cardiologist, Aseem Malhotra, is one of those doctors who has been talking about the problems with excess carbohydrates for some time. He also wrote in the *British Medical Journal* that saturated fat was not responsible for heart disease, but that these problems are instead driven by sugar and starchy foods such as bread, pasta, rice and potatoes. The article made international headlines.[16]

Cancer

Now that we can understand what insulin resistance is and how it plays a huge part in the development of obesity, type 2 diabetes and heart disease, we can also understand that it is most likely the root cause of many forms of cancer. Of course, there are many other causes we might have little or no control over but our lifestyle, stress levels and diet most likely affect the factors that allow cancer to grow. These factors are insulin (hyperinsulinaemia) and insulin-like growth factor (IGF), inflammation in the body and mitochondrial dysfunction.

Insulin-like growth factor is a hormone produced by the

liver. It acts very much like insulin. Its role is to control growth hormone secretion and so it promotes growth and the development of tissues. It is also involved in glucose metabolism, like insulin. Changes in IGF levels have been associated with hyperinsulinaemia, insulin resistance and diabetes, as well as the development and progression of cancer.[17, 18, 19]

Diabetes has been known to be connected with cancer for a long time, so it is obvious that insulin resistance is a problem that needs addressing when trying to prevent or treat cancer. Cancer cell metabolism requires high amounts of glucose, and it also benefits from fructose which increases the risk of more aggressive cancer.[20] Unlike healthy cells, which can use glucose, short-chain fatty acids (from fermenting fibre) or ketones as their energy source, , cancer cells are unable to use ketones for fuel. Ketones are formed from fat when following a diet very low in carbohydrate (page 75), A diet without sugar and low in other carbohydrates has therefore been said to starve those cancer cells while a diet high in sugar helps them to grow and spread. It is very likely that a high number of cancers could be prevented by diet, but also that a low-carb diet could help support good results during cancer treatment.

Cancer starts from a single cell. Such cells are probably being produced in our bodies all the time; it is thought that most people continually have tiny, microscopic cancer growths in their bodies, without these causing any harm. Our immune system recognises these bad cells and destroys them; we have a protective mechanism to stop them from growing any further.

For some reason, sometimes, these embryonic latent/potential cancer cells start to divide uncontrollably and won't stop, failing to respond to any normal growth-suppressing signals. They become immortal and could keep dividing forever. They ignore programmed cell death – apoptosis – that normal cells initiate when damaged. This dividing of cancer cells will eventually lead to the formation of cancer tumours. A growth like this then starts

Chapter 4

to form its own blood vessels in a process called 'angiogenesis', to supply it with oxygen and nutrients, making it possible for the cancer to grow and spread. Cancer cells can spread all over the body, an ability which will lead to metastases – secondary tumours. It seems that cancer cells also have the ability to defend themselves against the immune system, or avoid detection by it.

As I have said, cancer cells appear to use only sugar for energy. This is because their metabolism is very different from that of normal cells and they need a lot of glucose to produce energy – a lot more than normal cells. It seems that they are not that efficient at producing energy, possibly due to mitochondrial dysfunction. Cancer cells have been found to have abnormal mitochondria which do not function properly. For this reason, cancer has recently come to be seen more as a metabolic disease by some scientists, caused initially by mitochondrial dysfunction, rather than as a genetic disease.[21,22,23,24] This idea was first put forward by the Nobel Prize winner Otto Warburg in the early 1900s.

There are certain factors that cause the cancer to become more aggressive. One is sugar, as already explained, because it fuels cancer cells. The higher the blood glucose is, for example with diabetic patients, the worse the clinical prognosis and the more aggressive the cancer. Inflammation further encourages the development of cancer. We also know that factors supporting angiogenesis include hyperinsulinaemia, an unhealthy diet containing sugar, lack of nutrients, obesity, stress and smoking.

Cancer is able to grow when the circumstances are right. The problem with cancer treatment is that even when it is effective and destroys the cancer, there are almost always cancer cells left where the cancer started in the first place. If those circumstances which allowed the cancer to grow remain the same, it is very likely that the cancer will return and it often does so. We know that it is possible to treat cancer successfully – we have amazing treatments available today – but unfortunately for many patients, the cancer does return eventually. For this reason, lifestyle measures to support cancer treatment are extremely important.

Dementia and Alzheimer's disease

According to Alzheimer's Research UK, there are an estimated 850,000 people suffering from dementia in the UK. It has been estimated that by 2025 this number will have increased to one million. Globally there are an estimated 50 million people living with dementia, and this number is expected to triple by 2050.[25] The most common cause of dementia is Alzheimer's disease – according to the World Health Organization, it is probably responsible for 60-70% of dementia cases.

As we are all aware, Alzheimer's disease affects a person's memory, thinking (cognition) and behaviour, with progressive deterioration reducing the ability to perform everyday activities and live independently. This is why it is one of the biggest causes of disability and dependency around the world. It mainly affects older people – those aged 65 and above – but it does also occur in people aged 40-65. Even though most patients are elderly, it is very important to be aware that Alzheimer's disease is not a part of a normal aging. Many symptoms of insulin resistance are also listed as risk factors for Alzheimer's disease; these include obesity and type 2 diabetes. Smoking, excessive alcohol and lack of exercise are also risk factors for both. When looking at published research, it is clear that there is a connection between insulin resistance and Alzheimer's disease.[26, 27, 28, 29, 30, 31, 32, 33] This is why many scientists are calling Alzheimer's 'type 3 diabetes' – diabetes of the brain.

Insulin resistance seems to present differently in the brain compared with other parts of the body. It is known that insulin has a very important role in many functions in the brain – for example, in memory and cognition. There are insulin receptors at what is known as the 'blood–brain barrier' that protects the brain, as well as elsewhere in the brain. In areas involved in learning and memory, there are especially high numbers of these receptors; these areas include the hippocampus, the brain's memory centre. The development of Alzheimer's disease seems to be connected to problems with glucose metabolism in the brain which leads to damage in the nerve cells – the neurons – and eventually their death because they are unable to use glucose as fuel.

Problems with glucose metabolism in the brain lead to damaged nerve cells, initially in the hippocampus – the brain's memory centre

To enter the brain, insulin needs to cross the blood–brain barrier through these insulin receptors. It is these receptors that become resistant to insulin and consequently it becomes more difficult for insulin to enter the brain. Even if glucose is able to enter cells in the brain without insulin, they cannot process it and the brain cells are starved of fuel. Unlike other parts of the body, glucose can enter the brain through the blood–brain barrier, as well as into most brain cells, without insulin. In insulin resistance therefore there is lots of glucose in the brain, but deficient insulin, so the cells cannot process the glucose. High glucose levels are then constantly present in the brain, which damages the cells further. This is probably because of inflammation – as we already know, insulin resistance is associated with an inflammatory response elsewhere in the body. Accumulating glucose forms AGEs (as explained previously on page 18) which cause further damage. The first area to suffer is likely to be the hippocampus as it is such a metabolically active area and very sensitive to insulin deficits. This explains why problems with memory are the first signs of Alzheimer's disease, although it does eventually affect the whole brain.

This problem with glucose metabolism in the brain is called 'glucose hypometabolism'. It starts slowly and gradually becomes worse over the years as insulin resistance gets worse. The first changes happen decades before the symptoms but can be seen in PET scans.

Other brain/neurological problems

It seems that many other conditions affecting the brain also have an association with insulin resistance. Many of these are becoming more common, including depression. According to the World Health Organization, over 264 million people worldwide suffer from depression and it is increasingly affecting young people also.[34] There are many factors that can contribute to its development, including previous trauma or other life events in our past, but lifestyle issues, such as problems with the gut microbiome balance due to poor diet can contribute, as explained earlier in the book (page 26). The part insulin resistance plays in depression, anxiety and other mental problems is thought to be as follows.

In addition to the hippocampus, insulin is active in other important areas of the brain, with insulin receptors also seen in areas such as the hypothalamus. The hypothalamus regulates many functions in the body, including sleep, immune responses, many endocrine functions (hormonal balance) and sexual behaviour. It makes sense that problems with glucose metabolism, and also mitochondrial dysfunction due to chronic inflammation and oxidative stress, lead to many problems in the normal functioning of these areas too.

There is absolutely no doubt that a diet of processed, sugary food, not only high in carbohydrates but also very low in natural fats, affects our brain more than we would think.

Eye problems: glaucoma and macular degeneration

Glaucoma is now a very commonly diagnosed condition. It affects the optic nerve and without treatment can lead to loss of vision. Many scientists see it as a neurodegenerative disease, a problem in the brain like Alzheimer's disease, rather than a disease of the eye. After all, the optic nerve and retina are a part of the brain/nervous system.

It is very likely that the consequences of insulin resistance affect this area of the nervous system in the same way as the rest of the brain. Mitochondrial dysfunction, in addition to other problems caused by insulin resistance, has been found to be the cause of the development of glaucoma also.[35, 36] Indeed, the condition has recently been called 'type 4 diabetes' by some scientists because they are seeing it as part of the same problem with insulin resistance as 'type 3 diabetes' – Alzheimer's disease.

There is evidence that **age-related macular degeneration** is also a complication of insulin resistance.[37, 38, 39, 40, 41] Age-related macular degeneration (AMD) is, like glaucoma, a common condition. It does not cause total blindness but it affects the middle part of the sufferer's vision. However, it often gets worse without proper treatment. The exact cause is unclear, but it looks like metabolic dysfunction with oxidative stress and inflammation are causes of harm to the retina. The retina is also, like the optic nerve, extremely vulnerable to damage, being one of the most metabolically active tissues in the body.

Diabetic retinopathy is a well known complication of diabetes. It is very similar to AMD and those diabetic patients with retinopathy are also at a higher risk of developing AMD.[42] Diabetic retinopathy damages the small blood vessels in the retina. The root causes are the same as in AMD and glaucoma – insulin resistance and inflammation.

Summarising the consequences of insulin resistance

Because of insulin's multiple roles, insulin resistance can lead to a host of seemingly unrelated problems. These include:
- Problems with hormone balance, including PCOS, over/underactive thyroid, adrenal disorders, benign prostate enlargement and gynaecomastia
- Mouth and dental problems
- Osteoporosis/poor bone health
- Bowel problems, including IBS and IBD
- Chronic pain and associated conditions, including endometriosis, fibromyalgia and CFS/ME
- Peripheral neuropathy
- Gout
- Type 2 diabetes
- Heart disease
- Cancer
- Dementia and Alzheimer's disease owing to glucose hypometabolism in the brain
- Eye problems: glaucoma and macular degeneration.

Whether you have any of these problems already or think of them as 'in the family' it is never too soon to begin to reverse insulin resistance.

Chapter 5

How can I reverse insulin resistance?

We have excellent modern medicine and healthcare, with brilliant inventions in medications, for example. These treat acute health problems with amazing results. However, no medication is going to fix an underlying problem caused by insulin resistance. I personally think that most medicines, although they provide relief for acute problems, should not be used in the long term. Antacid medication is a good example of this; many people take such drugs for years, but wouldn't it be a lot easier and healthier to try to fix the cause of the symptoms with dietary measures? The possible side effects, many of them common, can be difficult to manage. For example, long-term antacid medication can cause changes in the gut microbiome. Many of us clinicians don't think about these problems when we write prescriptions, and many patients don't even want to know about them when they are looking for relief from their symptoms.

Chronic symptoms are almost always caused by something in our lifestyle, so we should at least look at the possible root causes before making decisions about long-term medication. The side effects of different medications might not matter so much with short-term courses, but what about years of regularly taking a medicine? Of course long-term medication has an effect on our body – statins are a common example. We know that mitochondria are often affected by certain medications and statin-associated muscle disease is understood to be caused by mitochondrial dysfunction, although the exact mechanism is not known. It is important always at least to try lifestyle changes first.

Whatever chronic health problem we have, a healthy diet is always the place to start

It does not matter what health condition or symptoms we suffer from, a good, healthy diet is always the first thing we have to think about when starting treatment. As we have seen, insulin resistance is a metabolic problem caused mostly by too much carbohydrate and sugar in our diet. Therefore, the first and the most important change in getting better is to fix that. This means we need to reduce the amount of sugar and carbohydrate we eat. As discussed earlier, excess weight and obesity are only symptoms of this metabolic problem as are other chronic conditions they are not the cause. It is completely illogical to think that by eating fewer calories, or exercising more, we could fix this. We can't. Unfortunately, however, these measures could potentially lead to even more complex problems in the long run.

Nutrition from our food is needed for everything in our body, from growth and repair – the formation of cells and cell membranes, bone marrow, blood and hormones – to keeping the body functioning properly. We really are what we eat. This is why, in addition to focusing on sugar and insulin, we need to make sure to eat good-quality, nutritious, 'real' (as opposed to processed) food full of the micronutrients we require. By choosing the right food we keep all our body functions working well and we stay healthy with a strong immune system.

Food matters a great deal, but so does our mind. Our mind also has an incredible power to help us heal even with the most difficult illnesses, such as cancer. We need to try to find ways to

Chapter 5

manage our stress, enjoy life and stay positive. We need to get out into the fresh air, enjoy nature, exercise and keep ourselves fit. We also need to make sure we get enough rest and sleep well, or as much as we possibly can.

When starting a new lifestyle, it is important not to make it too complicated. This helps us to avoid stress. For some people the only way to start a new lifestyle is to completely change their diet over one day, whereas for others it is best to take one step at a time, slowly making any changes. Whatever works best, it is important to listen to your body, but try to remember why you are doing this (to reverse insulin resistance) as this will help you stick to your new plan. The best food to eat is simple food; cook from basic ingredients, from scratch, simple dishes – for example, pan-fried fish with some steamed non-starchy vegetables and olive oil is easy and quick to cook and it makes a good meal. Try to plan your daily meals around those foods you usually like to eat, only leave all the starchy food and sugar out and enjoy a variety of veg with natural fat instead. Learn to cook yourself if you don't cook already.

Plan your daily meals around foods you like to eat only leave out the starchy foods and sugar

I also find that it is important to have support from family and/or friends and that they know why you are making these changes in your lifestyle. That way it is much easier to keep on going with your new way of living. If someone is willing to start this journey with you, even better.

Key actions

These are the key things you need to do to reverse insulin resistance. We will look at each in detail, one by one:
- Eat a diet low in carbohydrates

- Cut out sugar completely
- Don't eat more than three times per day and try intermittent fasting

In addition:
- Only eat good quality, real food
- Include lots of good, undamaged fats in your diet
- Keep your gut healthy
- Exercise
- Learn to manage stress
- Sleep well
- Do not smoke or vape
- Avoid alcohol.

Eat a diet low in carbohydrates

The benefits of a low-carbohydrate diet include:
- reduces the amount of insulin needed, resulting in a reduction of all symptoms caused by insulin resistance
- burns excess fat to reduce the harmful effects of fatty liver
- reduces chronic inflammation in the body effectively and boosts the immune system.

The aim with a low-carbohydrate diet is to keep insulin levels low, to prevent and treat insulin resistance. To be able to reduce the insulin in our body, we need to reduce the amount of carbohydrates we eat significantly, not just a little. Going back to 'Your metabolism' in Chapter 1 (page 1), you will remember that while we do need essential fatty acids and amino acids (from fats and proteins) in our diet, there are no essential carbohydrates. We also discussed how carbohydrates affect our blood glucose levels by causing them to rise, after which the pancreas responds by releasing insulin into our bloodstream to help transport the glucose into our cells. Carbohydrates are made up entirely of sugars and they all have this effect. Whether this sugar comes from fruit, a soft drink or bread, it will generally have the same effect on blood sugar and insulin levels. If we suffer from insulin resistance, we can only tolerate limited amounts of these foods.

A low-carbohydrate diet is sometimes referred to as a 'ketogenic diet' when the amount of carbohydrates we eat is very low. This is because, when following a diet low in carbohydrate, there is not much sugar for fuel and so the body switches to using fat instead. The liver produces ketone molecules from the fat we eat, or from our stored body fat. Our body can efficiently use ketones as an alternative fuel to produce energy if glucose is not available. The body is then said to be 'in the state of ketosis', either because we are fasting, or because the amount of carbohydrates we are eating is very low. When our insulin levels go down as a result of a diet low in carbohydrates, the opposite hormone to insulin, glucagon, is active, burning stored fat. As a result, we lose weight if we suffer from an excess. Our blood sugar levels stay stable, so we are less hungry, which increases our chances of losing weight effectively, if we need to. Because our insulin levels stay low, our symptoms start to get better.

Many people find that even the symptoms of autoimmune diseases, such as rheumatoid arthritis or asthma, improve, often very significantly, after reducing the amount of carbohydrate in their diet. This is probably because of the effect a diet low in carbohydrates has on inflammation. A ketogenic diet in particular has been found to be powerful in reducing inflammation in the body,[1, 2, 3, 4, 5, 6] providing of course that the diet is a 'real food' diet and does not contain refined oils, trans fats or other inflammatory foods. This results in a stronger immune system also; indeed, one study found a ketogenic diet to be effective against the influenza virus.[7] This study was done in mice, but it shows that a ketogenic diet is likely to have beneficial effects on immunity. In practice, many of my patients who follow a low-carb/ketogenic diet are very rarely unwell with a cold or a flu. The reason for their very strong immune system is no doubt their consumption of nutritious good food, but of course low insulin levels are important in reducing inflammation. A diet low in carbohydrate supports mitochondrial health, maintains ATP (energy) production better and reduces the generation of damaging/aging reactive oxygen species (ROSs). According to several studies, mitochondria are healthier and more viable when burning ketones as fuel.[8, 9, 10]

If you are a physically active person, even an athlete, it seems that ketones increase performance quite well, although there are different opinions about this. We will discuss what exercise to try on page 100.

Most of us simply cannot tolerate the amount of carbohydrates commonly-eaten food contains. Some people can tolerate more carbohydrates than others; it is usually easy to find your own 'limit' as you continue with low-carb eating. When you feel good and don't suffer from tiredness or cravings, you are likely to have found your ideal amount of carbohydrate. If you do suffer from hunger and cravings, you are probably eating too many carbohydrates. However, for someone who has a metabolic problem – insulin resistance – it is important that the daily amount of carbohydrate does not exceed 50 grams if the diet is to be effective in reducing the amount of insulin in the body. Some people need to cut down their carbohydrate intake even more than this. Many people with severe insulin resistance, or even type 2 diabetes, prefer a very strict diet and don't eat more than 20-30 g of carbohydrate a day.

What I have found is that you don't really need to measure the amount of carbohydrate you eat daily as such, as long as you avoid sugar and starchy foods. Please persevere with the diet. You will see extremely good results both mentally and physically, but remember that you cannot return to eating large amounts of carbs again, once you feel better. Insulin resistance is still there.

You will still be sensitive to excess amounts of sugar, and the symptoms will start to return if you ignore this.

> *Remember, you cannot return to eating large amounts of carbs once you feel better – insulin resistance is still there*

It is important to remember that if you suffer from insulin resistance, a low-carbohydrate diet is the lifestyle you need to follow for life, not a quick fix. Saying that, it is easy to follow because this type of lifestyle changes your whole relationship with food and eating. This is what many of my patients say too. Not only is the food delicious and very satisfying, but you don't feel that hungry ever, and you don't suffer from any cravings. You can take control of your eating, instead of food and cravings controlling you.

Cut out sugar completely

Cutting out sugar is a very important part of your new lifestyle. One of the best things to do to stay healthy for all of us is to give up sugar completely, and for anyone suffering from insulin resistance it is absolutely essential. This means giving up all sweets, cakes, biscuits, cereals and sugary drinks, and any other foods containing sugar, such as ketchup or salad dressings. Table sugar and sugar-like sweeteners, such as types of syrup, are extremely problematic and regular consumption will lead to ill health, sooner or later: as discussed earlier, sugar causes spikes in our insulin production which increase our risk of developing insulin resistance faster. It also affects our liver, causing fatty liver disease, as sugar is metabolised in the liver in the same way as alcohol; converted into fat, some of it stays in the liver if there is too much. This development again contributes to insulin resistance and certainly makes existing insulin resistance worse. Sugar is also highly inflammatory and causes chronic inflammation throughout the body. There is also evidence that it affects our gut microbiome, throwing it out of balance and thereby affecting our overall immunity.[11]

In my opinion, there is no 'safe' amount of sugar; no added sugar at all should be consumed in a healthy diet. As sugar is extremely addictive, for many of us, it is difficult to give it up, but many of my patients, and also I and my family, have learned to live without it, and we can see the health benefits clearly. Giving up sugar changes our palate also and soon foods that are sweet no longer taste that good. In fact, sugar only disguises other flavours – if there are any, which is probably why so many processed foods contain sugar; there really is no taste to processed foods without it.

'Natural' sweeteners, such as honey and maple syrup, are considered healthy and nutritious due to their micronutrient content but are of course also mostly sugar and contain high amounts of it, especially fructose. Although they can be consumed in small amounts by healthy, insulin-sensitive people, they should be avoided by anyone suffering from insulin resistance. The metabolic effects of them are exactly the same as sugar. This is the same for products like coconut sugar and agave syrup.

I never recommend any artificial sweeteners either. I don't believe such products can be a part of a healthy diet. There is also some evidence that sweeteners will keep the addiction to sweet foods going, and they can even affect insulin secretion.[12] Many of my patients have noticed this – consuming sweeteners causes cravings for sweet foods. There are also concerns about how some sweeteners affect our gut microbiome.[13] These are chemicals, not real food.

Avoid starchy food

A low-carbohydrate diet is a diet not only without any added sugar but also low in other sugary and starchy foods and drinks.

These starchy foods include bread, pasta, beans, rice, cereals, potatoes, sweet potatoes and drinks like beer. We often forget that sugar does not only mean added sugar but all carbohydrates are broken down into sugar in our body and they all have an effect on our blood sugar levels. In addition, sweet fruit such as bananas, grapes, mangos or pineapples, have the same effect and are too high in carbohydrate for anyone suffering from insulin resistance to tolerate. Root vegetables, although healthy in terms of fibre and micronutrients, contain more carbohydrates than vegetables that grow above the ground, so some caution with their consumption is advisable. Usually it is a good idea to avoid potatoes and sweet potatoes which are particularly high in carbohydrates. Beans are also quite high in carbohydrates, so not the best option for someone following a diet low in carbohydrate. (Green beans are not a problem.)

Avoid grains

Grains, also a starchy food, are often particularly difficult for many to cut out of their diet. Bread, pasta and cereals are such common foods, with so many of us eating them every day, often with every meal, but unfortunately, grains also break down to sugar; in fact, they are very high in carbohydrates, and not suitable for anyone suffering from insulin resistance. According to the sugar infographics published by the Public Health Collaboration,[14] just one serving of bread (30 grams), both white and brown, is equivalent to 3-4 teaspoons of table sugar. This would greatly affect blood sugar levels and cause insulin spikes. Many of my patients who have already cut out sugar, don't realise that grains are essentially the same thing when it comes to how they affect the blood sugar and insulin levels.

Grains can be very problematic food for many people, not only because of their carbohydrate content but also because of a condition called 'gluten sensitivity'. Gluten is a protein in grains. Coeliac disease is an autoimmune disease with gluten intolerance and patients suffering from coeliac disease are unable to tolerate any gluten in their diet. It seems though, that many people with no diagnosis of coeliac disease are still unable to consume foods containing gluten, such as bread or pasta. This condition has been called 'non-coeliac gluten sensitivity'. The symptoms of this usually include abdominal problems such as bloating, diarrhoea and constipation.

People with coeliac disease very often suffer from changes in their gut microbiome which can affect their overall immunity and lead to chronic inflammation, as discussed in Chapter 1. Even without coeliac disease, it is likely that gluten sensitivity will have a similar effect. Recurrent diarrhoea, for example, can affect the microbiome, but also interfere with the normal absorption of micronutrients.

If gluten is affecting the lining of our bowel, causing inflammation, the situation can lead to the development of leaky gut syndrome (see Chapter 2 – page 26); this is a situation where intestinal permeability increases, due to this inflammation, which leads to unwanted substances entering the bloodstream. This in turn can trigger autoimmune responses leading to chronic inflammation in the body getting worse, which will again cause insulin resistance, or make it worse.

One of the reasons many people are worried about whether they need grains or not is fibre. However, vegetables consumed in a low-carbohydrate diet, as well as berries, are in fact much higher in fibre than traditional whole-grain options such as bread. I often need to remind my patients of the fact that a low-carbohydrate diet is by no means a diet low in fibre. We eat plenty of delicious vegetables which in fact also offer much better nutritional value than do grains, even whole grains.

Be careful with drinks

It is important to remember that drinks can also cause insulin spikes in our body, so we must focus not only on what we eat, but also what we drink. Sweet sugary drinks are by far the worst drink choices but this does not only include sugary lemonade, or colas, but also fruit juices. Fruit juices are actually extremely high in sugar, with a 200 ml serving of pure apple juice affecting our blood sugar the same way as more than 8 teaspoons of sugar would (Public Health Collaboration UK, PHCUK, sugar infographics[14]). This is worth remembering also where children are concerned. When we eat fruit, we normally eat only one at a time while a glass of juice is likely to contain much more than this, increasing the amount of sugar we consume.

Water is absolutely the best drink on a low-carbohydrate diet. It keeps us well hydrated and has nothing added to it. Both still water and sparking water are great. If you prefer some more taste to the water, you can add lemon to it and also try adding fresh mint, or even some berries or fruit slices to give it a nice flavour.

Coffee and tea are also okay to drink but without any sugar or sweetener. One teaspoon of sugar contains 4 grams of carbohydrates,[14] so trying to keep within the daily limits of 50 grams of carbohydrates becomes difficult – it all adds up. Also be careful with large amounts of milk in your drink because of lactose, the sugar in milk. It is best to avoid it as much as possible. Cream contains a lot less carbohydrate than milk and might be a better option.

Many of us occasionally like to enjoy smoothies, or green juices, for their health benefits. Many of them can be a good way to start the day, but be careful with their sugar content. Smoothies that mainly contain fruit are usually very high in sugar and therefore cause problems with insulin resistance. However, a smoothie that mainly contains vegetables can be a good and healthy drink. Vegetables like spinach, avocado or cucumber are good ingredients in a smoothie, with only a few carbohydrates. On the other hand, berries are not that high in carbohydrates, so when used sensibly, add their lovely flavour to smoothies and other drinks. (See below for more on vegetables and berries but generally any vegetable, apart from beans, that grows above the ground will have a low-carbohydrate content. Fruit is another issue.)

Don't eat too often

If we follow these three rules we will end up eating less automatically, and this kind of a proper rhythm to eating also has a powerful balancing effect on our hormones:

- Don't eat more than three times per day
- Don't snack
- Try intermittent fasting

Our body needs time when we eat and collect nutrients and energy, and time when we don't eat but consume stored energy. All these functions are regulated by different hormones, as explained in Chapter 1. Eating too often, whether it is having too many meals a day or just small snacks, disturbs this balance. Every time we eat, insulin is needed whereas its opposite hormone, glucagon, cannot work efficiently. Eating too frequently results in too much insulin in the body all the time, which will make insulin resistance worse. Following a diet low in carbohydrates and eating only at meal times restores the correct balance of hormones very quickly and helps to reduce insulin resistance.

Eating too often disturbs the balance between the hormones insulin (which stores sugar) and glucagon (which takes sugar out of storage)

We need to eat well, until we are satisfied. It is important that we are not left hungry after our meals as this increases the risk of snacking. Eating a low-carbohydrate diet helps as it makes us less hungry; many people eating this way quickly notice that there is no need for any extra snacks. The main meals are very filling and keep us satisfied until the next meal.

Chapter 5

Intermittent fasting

The benefits of intermittent fasting include:
- quickly reduces excess sugar in the body in type 2 diabetes
- reduces insulin levels in the body
- reduces insulin resistance quickly and effectively, resulting in reduced symptoms caused by insulin resistance
- restores hormonal balance
- increases autophagy (cell spring cleaning) in mitochondria
- raises energy levels and improves concentration.

Intermittent fasting has recently become a popular and powerful intervention, especially for obesity and type 2 diabetes. It lowers insulin very efficiently and helps us to lose weight. With the three-meals-a-day rhythm recommended in low-carbohydrate eating, we automatically go through a longer fast every day anyway, depending on when we eat, but mostly overnight, between dinner and breakfast. This is ideal when preventing weight gain and when we don't suffer from significant insulin resistance. However, if there is a significant amount of weight to lose or difficult insulin resistance to reverse, including longer periods of fasting into the daily routine is very beneficial.

Fasting will help reduce insulin resistance quickly. Short-term intermittent fasting seems to be extremely good for our overall health,[15, 16, 17, 18, 19, 20, 21, 22, 23, 24, 25, 26, 27, 28, 29, 30, 31, 32, 33, 34, 35, 36, 37, 38] so it is worth trying even with less severe insulin resistance. It actually is the ancient secret of health; fasting has been practised throughout human history. And it still is.

There are several ways to include intermittent fasting in your daily routine. Some people fast for 20-24 hours one to three times a week and either fast all day, or only eat once – for example, just dinner on fasting days. Others fast for 16 hours on most days and eat only within an 8-hour window, usually lunch and dinner, but no breakfast.

When we are fasting (i.e. not eating) our metabolism, as explained in Chapter 1, functions in reverse. Our insulin levels drop quickly and when this happens, our body burns stored energy, first stored glycogen which is broken down into glucose and used as energy. Then, as we are not getting any more sugar in, after the glycogen stores have been used, our body switches to burning stored fat. This means intermittent fasting has many benefits. Fasting effectively burns all excess sugar in the body and it lowers insulin levels fast. This makes it very powerful in reversing even difficult insulin resistance quickly, especially if we suffer from type 2 diabetes with raised blood sugar levels. The body then uses ketones as fuel very effectively and we feel more energetic.

Fasting also increases the amount of growth hormone naturally which further helps in burning extra fat, especially around the midriff; it also helps us to gain muscle and preserve lean muscle. Growth hormone typically goes down with age and very low levels in older people may lead to lower muscle and bone mass. This benefit – that we lose fat only, not muscle – is also a benefit of a ketogenic diet. It is also important to note that fasting does not cause any of the adverse side effects which are associated with excessive growth hormone when artificial growth hormones are used.

Intermittent fasting also stimulates **autophagy**, the cleaning process in cells discussed in Chapter 1. This process is essential for our health and it is important to be aware that the modern way of eating too often and snacking actually reduces this process and thereby obstructs the 'renewal' system of the body.

Intermittent fasting also reduces inflammation in the body, not only because of reduced sugar and insulin levels, but also because it protects our body against oxidative stress. This will

help reverse insulin resistance even further. When fasting:
- don't consume any calorie-containing food or drink
- remember to drink enough water – at least 2 litres a day.

You can have tea or coffee if you like, but of course with no sugar or other sweeteners, and be wary of milk. I normally also enjoy green tea and various herbal teas, such as peppermint.

Remember that if you feel hungry during fasting, it will soon pass. You won't be constantly hungry; this feeling comes and goes. As your body gets more used to fasting and starts to burn your fat stores, you will feel less and less hungry. Generally, intermittent fasting is a lot easier for people already following a diet low in carbohydrates. This is because they are never that hungry anyway and don't suffer from any cravings. It is okay to skip a meal if necessary.

Caution: Please remember that people with certain medical conditions, such as type 1 diabetes, should not attempt fasting without strict medical supervision. Pregnant or breastfeeding women and people who are underweight or underage, should not fast either. If in any doubt, it is a good idea to consult your doctor.

Eat only good quality, real food

It is very important to eat good quality food when following a diet that is low in carbohydrates and/or ketogenic. It is all about good nutrition for our body. It is important to focus on micronutrients and eat plenty of organic vegetables, herbs, berries, spices and other nutritious foods. Our body needs a variety of micronutrients for its many functions – for example, we know that our mitochondria depend on many micronutrients and lack of these causes problems with our energy production – something we don't really think about that much. Vitamins and other micronutrients will also help in reducing inflammation and support our bowel health. Although we may additionally need some supplements to support our health, the most important thing is to make sure we eat well.

I do often recommend supplements to my patients who suffer from insulin resistance, in addition to healthy food. Most commonly these are vitamin D3, vitamin C and magnesium.[39, 40, 41, 42, 43, 44, 45, 46, 47, 48]

Vitamin D3 is essential for many functions in our body, including our immune response. It is also thought to improve insulin sensitivity and it has a role in regulating insulin production. Deficiency is unfortunately very common, especially amongst people suffering from insulin resistance, and it increases the risk of complications. It is very important to ensure you have sufficient levels. Sunlight is the main and best source of vitamin D and dietary sources are often not sufficient, especially during the winter months, so supplementation is necessary.

Vitamin C: Many patients might also benefit from vitamin C supplementation, especially if their dietary vitamin C intake has been poor in the past, they find that their immunity is low and/or they also smoke. There is evidence also that vitamin C helps in reducing insulin resistance due to its antioxidant properties.

Magnesium: This mineral is important for normal insulin activity and deficiency has been found to be common in people with insulin resistance. Magnesium supplementation can improve insulin sensitivity and help to reduce insulin resistance.

Other supplements might be beneficial in reducing inflammation as well as restoring health. However, any possible deficiencies are very different in different people, therefore please consult a knowledgable doctor or functional nutritionist.

Eat plenty of vegetables and herbs

The only carbohydrates that we need every day are vegetables, particularly for their nutritional content. For all the important micronutrients, it is advisable to eat many different varieties, including different cabbages, kale, spinach, fennel, courgette, bell peppers, cucumber, cauliflower and mushrooms.

If you have a problem with insulin resistance, it is important always to remember not to cause extra stress to your body with too many carbohydrates, so the best vegetables to consume are those that grow above the ground; they are naturally low in carbohydrates and, because of this, can be eaten freely when following a diet low in carbohydrate.

It is also very important to use lots of different herbs for their vitamin content as well as other highly nutritious foods, such as ginger, garlic, turmeric and many other spices.

Try to avoid cooked root vegetables in larger quantities as they tend to contain quite a lot of starch. If you like to eat carrots or beetroot, for example, it is better to eat them raw or only very gently cooked and in smaller quantities. When suffering from insulin resistance, eating any foods containing high amounts of starch – glucose ultimately – including potatoes, will add to our problems with insulin and slow down our recovery.

My dietary recommendations for my patients usually include those vegetables that I know to be particularly healthy, nutrition-rich foods. These are spinach, kale, fresh herbs such as parsley and coriander, broccoli, ginger, garlic, cabbage, including red cabbage, Brussels sprouts and carrots (raw). The micronutrients and antioxidants that these foods contain help to lower inflammation in the body, support mitochondrial function and provide good fibre to help keep our gut microbiome in balance.

Avoid most fruit, choose berries

It is best not to eat much fruit as all fruit naturally contains a lot of sugar, which in large amounts is harmful – as discussed earlier – and again makes existing insulin resistance worse. And if you are trying to lose weight, or suffer from diabetes, it is best to avoid most fruit altogether. The situation is the same as with root vegetables – most types of fruit are nutritious but, if we suffer from insulin resistance, the sugar content in them can be too much for our body to cope with. If you like fruit, it is best to eat local apples or plums, in small amounts, when in season. They contain much less sugar compared with many other fruits, such as bananas or grapes, for example. Melons also contain much less carbohydrate and are okay to eat in small quantities.

Berries are a much better choice; I always recommend including berries in a diet generally low in carbohydrate. They contain much less carbohydrate compared with other types of fruit and are packed with micronutrients and antioxidants – indeed, their micronutrient content is higher than fruit like bananas. Berries are actually considered one of the healthiest foods we can eat for this reason. This antioxidant content reduces oxidative stress and inflammation in the body. This might be the reason why some studies have also found berries to improve our insulin sensitivity.[49, 50, 51, 52]

Choose good quality protein, preferably organic

Protein is very important for our body. We need essential amino acids from good protein sources for our immune function, to build and repair cell membranes and tissues, to produce hormones and enzymes, and for mitochondrial activity. However, regular advice has been that if you suffer from insulin resistance and/or are trying to lose weight, you should keep the amount of protein you eat at a moderate level. A low-carbohydrate diet is not meant to be a 'high-protein diet' instead. This is because too much protein can also cause spikes in insulin levels. This in turn can cause extra strain on the liver and increase insulin resistance, because the liver converts excess protein to glucose via gluconeogenesis (the process explained on page 49). Saying that, there are many different views on how much this process affects our blood glucose and insulin levels. Some studies suggest not much at all,[53, 54] and the effect protein has on insulin levels also depends on our overall carbohydrate intake and our metabolic health. It seems that it is much better to ensure we are getting an adequate amount of protein from our diet than to worry about getting too much and then increase the risk of deficiency in vital amino acids.

How much protein?

So protein is an essential part of our diet, but the amount we need depends on our age and activity level. It is important to remember that our body's ability to break down protein into amino acids reduces as we get older so we need to eat more protein to preserve our muscle mass and prevent a condition called sarcopenia – age-related muscle loss.

As explained above, there is debate about exactly how much protein we need. We know that in addition to the elderly, growing children also need more good quality protein than adults and also, if we exercise a lot, or we are unwell, recovering from an illness or perhaps an operation, our protein needs are raised. It seems that for most of us the recommended intake is generally around 1.2-1.8 g of protein per kg of body weight per day, or approximately 25-35 g of protein per meal. It is difficult of course to keep measuring the amount of protein we eat with each meal, but as a rough guide this amount usually equals 1-2 fillets of fish, a moderate portion of meat/chicken or 2-3 eggs per meal, for example.

It is important to eat until satisfied, but not to overeat, and to keep an eye on our portion sizes while remembering that insulin resistance is a problem caused by too much carbohydrate, not protein. When we manage to reverse insulin resistance and restore our hormonal and metabolic balance, we don't suffer from addictions and never overeat. It is easier to keep our food portions at a level suitable for our body.

Sources of protein

When choosing protein to eat, again, it is important to remember to go for real food. Many of the processed protein bars and powders marketed to boost our fitness are not only completely unnecessary but are also unlikely to be healthy. Look for good, natural sources of protein: eggs, fermented dairy such as cheese and yoghurt, nuts, free-range meat, poultry and wild fish. These are all extremely healthy foods and, in addition to good quality protein, they provide us with many essential micronutrients and fatty acids – all important for normal body functions.

Dairy, if you can tolerate it well, is a good source of protein, but it contains lactose – milk sugar. For that reason it is important to avoid large amounts of milk, in particular, and to use only moderate amounts if needed, for example in coffee or tea. It is good to notice though that cream contains far less carbohydrate compared to milk and can be a better alternative. Another important issue to note is that fermented dairy products, such as cheese, butter, yoghurt and kefir, are not only very healthy, but usually well tolerated by those who cannot tolerate milk as such. Fermented dairy is rich in omega-3 fatty acids and another essential fatty acid called CLA – conjugated linoleum acid. It also contains vitamin K2 – essential for our heart health.

Fat is a vital part of our diet. We will discuss dietary fat in the next chapter (page 94), but it is worth mentioning here that a low-carbohydrate diet is all about real food that is low in sugar; not about reducing fat. For that reason, always choose good quality dairy, as unprocessed as possible to ensure proper nutrients. Processed low-fat or fat-free products don't belong in a healthy diet.

Nuts are known to contain lots of healthy fatty acids as well as good quality fibre. Include them in your diet in moderation (this means a handful of nuts a day). Choose Brazils, pecans, macadamias, walnuts, almonds, pine nuts and hazelnuts. Be a little more careful with cashews and pistachio nuts as they are significantly higher in carbohydrates. It is okay to add some spices and salt if you like, but avoid vegetable oils. Raw nuts are a better option than roasted as roasting can damage nut fats.

Free range meat and poultry, like eggs and fish, offer an excellent source of complete protein. They also contain many important micronutrients, including iron, zinc and vitamin B_{12}. In addition, there are many other important compounds in meat that are considered very healthy and extremely beneficial when reversing insulin resistance and restoring health. These include:

- the amino acid carnosine with anti-inflammatory, immune-strengthening properties
- glutathione, which supports mitochondrial health
- choline, a vital nutrient for our nervous system and cognitive functions
- coenzyme Q10, which is extremely important for healthy functioning of mitochondria.[55, 56, 57, 58, 59]

These are only example of how important it is to know what it is we are eating. I explained in Chapter 1 how there are very many micronutrients that are essential for mitochondria health and functioning.

Red meat such as lamb is very rich in these nutrients. It contains omega-3 fatty acids, oleic acid (the primary fat also in olive oil), lots of different B-group vitamins, especially vitamin B_{12}, zinc and selenium.

Poultry such as goose is also an excellent source of dietary glycine, an amino acid needed for the synthesis of collagen (very important for our skin health, but it also has a role in metabolic processes and might help in inflammatory conditions such as osteoarthritis). This amino acid is often low in people who suffer from insulin resistance.[60] There are also many vital minerals such as iron, selenium and zinc.

Organ meat (liver, kidneys, sweetbreads) is also extremely

rich in nutrients; in addition to coQ10, it is rich in vitamins A and B$_{12}$ as well as many minerals.

It is advisable to avoid processed meat such as low-quality sausages or bacon. They usually contain many additives, including nitrites, and it is also very difficult to find any bacon, salami, ham or other similar foods without added sugar.

Fish, especially fatty fish, that is wild-caught, such as mackerel or sardines, is highly nutritious and one of the healthiest foods you can eat. Fish contains particularly healthy fats and fatty fish is an excellent source of omega-3 fatty acids in their best and most bioavailable forms of EPA and DHA (please also see page 95), many micronutrients and high quality protein.

Eggs are also an excellent source of good quality protein and contain many important micronutrients, including vitamin B$_{12}$ and other B group vitamins; also vitamin D. Eggs are also a rich source of choline and selenium.

If you don't eat meat or fish, that is absolutely fine too. It is perfectly possible to follow a vegetarian diet that is low in carbohydrates. The main problem with many vegetarian diets with regard to insulin resistance has been the fact that they often consist of large amounts of grains, legumes, pulses and starchy vegetables, all of which are very high in carbohydrates. However, if you eat eggs and dairy, or fermented soy products such as tofu or tempeh, it is easy to follow this diet. Seeds such as hemp seeds and many nuts are also high in protein and healthy fats, and low in carbohydrates.

Avoid processed food

We have discussed the problems chronic inflammation causes, from whole-body to cellular level. It is important to try to reduce inflammation by avoiding foods that cause it, such as sugar, or starchy carbs and refined oils. Processed food often contains pro-inflammatory ingredients, such as sugar, excess salt, trans fats (see below), sulphites and nitrites. In addition, carbohydrate content can be too high for someone with insulin resistance. For example, many ready-meals contain high amounts of carbohydrates and no natural fat.

We often forget that the way to a good healthy life can be very simple. Common sense will probably tell you that the less processed food you eat, the better. If your lunch box today contains a fillet of mackerel with some salad or low-carb vegetables, and extra virgin olive oil, for example, it will make you feel good, you will be able to do all the things you were planning to do and your mind will stay sharp. Furthermore, you will be satisfied until dinner time without any need for snacks. If you eat a ready-made lunch, heated up in a microwave oven, or a sandwich made with processed bread and a packet of crisps, you will almost certainly be tired and lethargic at some point and not want to continue with your day. You will feel hungry again after a few hours and need a snack, and possibly another one before your dinner. You'll end up eating too much and too often. We've all been there.

Many processed foods, and especially ultra-processed foods, are also lacking in nutrients essential for our health. Refining, pasteurising, homogenising, genetically modifying and using chemicals or pesticides all alter foods in ways that reduce nutrition with potentially devastating effects. Many of these methods destroy most of the benefits of the original foods and turn them into something completely different. Compare, for example, unpasteurised, full-fat cheese with a reduced-fat, processed variety. One contains healthy fatty acids and numerous enzymes and nutrients to benefit our bodies. The other contains damaged fats, few vitamins and no enzymes.

Pesticides: There is also evidence that certain pesticides used in modern farming can cause stress in the body and affect our bowel health, leading to leaky gut syndrome (page 28) and increasing inflammation. Levels of these are particularly high in GM foods as they are modified to resist pesticides selectively.

My advice would therefore be to buy only basic ingredients and prepare all your food yourself and always choose organic and free-range products whenever possible. These are healthier, free of pesticides and much better for the environment too. By eating real food you can make sure that you and your family get many important nutrients from what you eat and you will also prevent the inflammation behind many health problems, including insulin resistance.

Choose natural fats and avoid refined oils and margarines

As I explained in Chapter 2 (page 20), it is important not to eat refined oils and margarines to avoid or reduce existing inflammation. They are damaged fats and, if used in our body in place of natural fats, can disrupt cell membranes and their functioning. We also need to remember to restore a better balance between omega-6 and omega-3 essential fatty acids. As explained earlier, this should be between 4:1 and 1:1, depending on which experts you listen to.

We know that fat has an extremely important part in a healthy diet. We can burn saturated fats for fuel in place of carbohydrates and cholesterol is the precursor for many hormones, including the sex hormones testosterone, oestrogen and progesterone. We also need fat/oil for the absorption of the fat-soluble vitamins A, D, E and K.

When we have natural fat in out diet, we ensure we have access to all these important micro-nutrients, but food that contains enough fat is also delicious and keeps us full and satisfied longer. It is easier not to snack. Fat does not have any effects on our blood sugar levels or insulin production either. We thereby reduce inflammation and insulin resistance.

'Healthy fats' mean natural fats, which include butter, cheese, fatty fish, goose fat and other animal-based fats, extra-virgin coconut oil (and other coconut products), nuts and extra-virgin olive oil. Also cacao is healthy, so as long as you are careful with any sugar content: small amounts of very dark chocolate or raw chocolate (or cocoa powder) are actually very good for you. They contain a high level of polyphenols – the plant chemicals that can boost our health.

Extra-virgin olive oil in particular is one of the healthiest foods we can have in our diet and so makes a good basis for our natural fat intake, though it is important to note that sufficient omega-6 and omega-3 fatty acids must come from other sources. It is known to reduce inflammation and improve markers of metabolic disease, such as HDL cholesterol. It tastes lovely with vegetables, but I have also learned that – contrary to what I had previously thought – it is also a very stable cooking fat.[101] Olive oil mostly contains monounsaturated fat which makes it less prone to oxidation compared to polyunsaturated fats such as sunflower oil. Although it is not as stable as saturated fat, it contains protective antioxidants which possibly increase resistance to oxidation.

In addition to extra virgin olive oil, as already mentioned when discussing proteins, fatty fish is an important part of a healthy diet because of the EPA and DHA fatty acids that it contains. The best vegetarian sources of omega-6 and omega-3 fats include linseed/flaxseed, at a ratio of roughly 4:1 – but not linseed oil as the extraction process for seed oils is damaging. It is important to notice though that although the body converts the plant-based omega-3 fatty acid, alpha-linolenic acid (ALA) into EPA and DHA fatty acids, this is only to a very limited extent.

Keep your gut healthy

As explained earlier in the book, a healthy gut is extremely important in preventing any illness as the micro-organisms in our gut (collectively, the microbiome) have an important role in our immune system and the control of inflammation. As we have seen, chronic inflammation goes hand in hand with insulin resistance, with each exacerbating the other.

Dietary measures discussed in this chapter will help to treat a possible imbalance in the gut microbiome. This might take some time, as the microbiome cannot recover overnight from possibly years of eating an unhealthy diet, but there will be improvement every day. The time it takes for the balance to be restored varies from person to person. It depends on the situation in the gut. If you suffer from leaky gut syndrome, it will take longer to recover, so it is important to be persistent with the measures recommended here. However, the composition of the microbiome changes quickly, which will help.

Probiotics and prebiotics

To maintain a healthy gut, we need both probiotics and prebiotics. Fermented products contain probiotics – bacteria that are beneficial to our gut, such as *Lactobacillus acidophilus*. These have actually always been part of a healthy diet in many parts of the world. Fermentation has been used as a natural way to prevent food from going off with no refridgeration available. Natural fermentation – lactofermentation – is a process which preserves the food and all its nutrients, and creates many beneficial enzymes, B vitamins, omega-3 fatty acids, vitamin K2 and many different strains of probiotic. Fizzy drinks used to be made by fermentation also. Good old-fashioned ginger beer is a great example of this. Many delicious fermented foods like sauerkraut (fermented cabbage) or kimchi (fermented vegetables), are still widely used in many cultures even though they are not so well known in the UK or America anymore. However, many people have become more aware of the benefits of fermented food and drink and these products are now common in many health stores and increasingly in supermarkets too.

Chapter 5

It is highly beneficial to regularly consume fermented products as they are full of healthy pro-biotics. Even just a few spoonfuls a day are enough to provide you with millions of good, protective bacteria to look after your gut. In my family, we try to make these fermented foods ourselves. It is quite easy to do once you get the hang of it. I have included a sample recipe at the end of the book (page 133). You can also try natural yoghurt or kefir as well as unpasteurised cheese, kombucha drink or miso for the same benefits.

In addition to avoiding sugar and introducing fermented products into your diet, certified probiotic supplements might also help in some cases. Products containing different strains of bacteria, such as *Lactobacillus acidophilus*, *Bifidobacterium bifidum* and *Bifidobacterium lactis* are often recommended as they have been shown to reduce imbalances in our microbiome caused by inflammation or infection and may even heal leaky gut syndrome.[61, 62, 63] Also in cases where we have had to have a course of antibiotics for treatment of a bacterial infection, these probiotics have been found to reduce problems such as diarrhoea caused by the medication.

Along with probiotics, we are also advised to make sure we eat enough gut-microbiome-friendly foods called prebiotics. Prebiotics are foods – mainly vegetables – containing types of soluble fibre that provide nutrition for the microbiome. This is mainly in the form of oligosaccharides in berries and apples as well as vegetables such as cabbage, broccoli, leeks, onions, garlic, and asparagus, which are fermented by the gut flora to form short chain fatty acids. A low-carbohydrate diet, containing real food and plenty of vegetables, is therefore an ideal way of eating to maintain a healthy gut.

Ensuring enough omega-3 in the diet is also important as these fatty acids too act as beneficial prebiotics.[68]

Homemade stock from bones is also worth mentioning as a gut-friendly food. It contains gelatin/collagen with many important amino acids, such as proline and glycine. These are important in supporting a healthy gut lining and function.[64]

FODMAPs

If you suffer from any abdominal symptoms which continue after starting a sugar-free diet low in carbohydrate and containing probiotics and prebiotics, it is important to look at other possible causes for the symptoms. In addition to gluten (non-coeliac gluten sensitivity, page 80) some other components in food might cause problems. For example, not consuming foods con-taining fermentable oligo-, di- or mono-saccharides and polyols (FODMAPs) has helped many people suffering from abdominal discomfort. Common FODMAPs are fructose, lactose, fructans, galactans and polyols. They are short-chain carbohydrates, which cause problems for some people. Fructose is found in many fruit and vegetables, lactose in dairy products such as milk, fructans in grains, galactans in legumes and polyols in many sweeteners, fruits and vegetables. They are fermented by bacteria in the colon, and produce smelly hydrogen gas and cause digestive symptoms in some people. According to studies, many people with IBS symptoms might have problems with FODMAPs.[99, 100]

Because maintaining a healthy gut is vital in reversing insulin resistance and reducing inflammation, it is advisable to try eliminating FODMAPs from the diet if abdominal symptoms continue.

Other actions to support a healthy gut

> **Avoid additives:** Avoid anything processed in your diet to maintain bowel health. Many additives can cause problems in the bowel microbiome. Carrageenan, for example, is used to thicken or emulsify many foods,

including some nut milks and yoghurts. There are a lot of worries about how carrageenan can potentially cause inflammation in the bowel. Although clearly more research is needed in this area, my advice would be to avoid any unnecessary additives.

Minimise antibiotic use: Commonly used antibiotics can also be harmful to the balance of our gut. Remember to try to avoid antibiotics unless they are absolutely necessary – they will not help with viral infections such as colds and flu. Unnecessary antibiotics can cause imbalance in your gut for a long time which will in turn have an impact on your overall health.

Manage stress: Good stress management is very important for bowel health too. As discussed previously, chronic stress causes many abdominal symptoms via the gut–brain connection; it can also upset the balance of the gut microbiome. This works the other way too; you can significantly reduce stress and other psychological symptoms by looking after your gut health. I look at ways to manage stress on page 102.

Exercise has also been scientifically proven to increase the amount, and diversity, of beneficial gut bacteria.[65, 66, 67]

In summary, to ensure a healthy gut, include the following foods in your diet:
- fermented foods and probiotics
- prebiotics (soluble fibre)
- omega-3 fatty acids[68]
- homemade bone stock.

In addition to dietary measures:
- avoid unnecessary medication

- remember stress management
- take regular exercise.

Exercise regularly

A low-carb diet together with exercise burns fat very efficiently, but also develops muscles. Any kind of exercise we enjoy has positive benefits for us, but there are some studies that show that 'high intensity interval training' (HIIT – see below), in particular, is very good for improving insulin sensitivity in the cells.[69, 70]

HIIT has recently become very popular with people interested in low-carbohydrate eating. It seems to be a much better alternative than traditional long-distance jogging and it has a much greater effect on insulin levels. I have also found it to be extremely beneficial for aerobic and cardiovascular fitness, and in much less time than is normally used in endurance training. HIIT has also been shown to release exercise-induced growth hormone, which makes it very efficient at strength building and fat burning and for anti-aging. HIIT, like exercise generally, increases the number of mitochondria and improves mitochondrial respiration. It helps you gain muscle fast which increases your metabolism, improves oxygen consumptions significantly and is very good for your heart health. It also effectively reduces stress by lowering those stress hormone levels. These are all extremely important factors when treating insulin resistance.

The idea of HIIT is to repeat a certain movement with varying levels of intensity, starting with a slow movement, followed by short period of intense, fast exercise, such as sprinting. When outdoors, for example, you can start with walking and, during the fast interval, continue with maximum speed or weight, for only 20-30 seconds. After that you return to walking again to calm your pulse and breathing. Typically this type of exercise lasts from 10 to 30 minutes. The length of the exercise, and the rest, periods depend on your fitness level. In addition to doing HIIT outdoors, there are other options too, especially if you enjoy fitness classes. For example, dancing or cross-fit training are both very good options, and great fun. Tabata training combines intensity intervals of cardio and strength training also and is very beneficial.

As I have said, HIIT is a very effective way to reduce insulin resistance when combined with a low-carb diet. It does not matter how fit or unfit you are, or how old you are when starting, you can do the exercise completely at your own pace. For maximum benefits you can combine HIIT with some form of strength training, including simple pull ups, push-ups, squats and planks, to strengthen your muscles.

Walking, hiking and cycling are also good ways to keep fit and reduce stress, as well as for socialising if you have someone to go with. Nothing beats a good conversation while walking, for example, although I do sometimes enjoy walks on my own also. When walking or hiking in nature – in the woods, over the fields or on the beach – you will find you can do HIIT-type spurts naturally, going up a hill or across more difficult/heavy terrain. Exercise is extremely beneficial in reducing stress, especially if done out of doors, rather than in a gym. It is free, but I and my family also find walking in nature has an incredibly calming effect on us. We love to go out together for long walks at least once a week. This gives us a great opportunity to spend time together and have some good conversations. So, it is not just the physical benefits of exercise that are important, but also the psychological.

Another form of exercise we also enjoy as a family is gardening, which can be a type of HIIT exercise too, with lifting, lawn mowing or digging involved.

Personally, I also very much enjoy yoga. It gives a lovely balance in addition to HIIT exercise. Yoga is a calming form of exercise, often including meditation, breathing exercises and poses designed to help with relaxation. In contrast to other types of yoga, which are all good in their different ways, yin specifically calms the mind, relaxes and stretches the body. It helps to increase flexibility and strength and increases one's energy levels. It is the perfect way to relax in the middle of our busy lives, which is why I recommend it to many of my patients. The many benefits of yoga have been backed by science,[71, 72] so it is ideal alongside other ways of treating insulin resistance. Yoga increases physical strength, but it is its effect on psychological wellbeing and the immune system (via the gut–brain axis) that is thought to be why it is a good method when treating insulin resistance.

Learn to manage stress

In primary care clinics it is shocking to see how many people today are battling with depression, anxiety and other mental health problems. Many of them are young people, some even children. There are many reasons for these problems, including the demands of our busy modern life. Worries about studies, work, finances and grief for loved ones all cause great stress. However, it is clear that the wrong food and a poor lifestyle are very often the root cause of mental problems. Sugar and processed foods especially affect the mind in many ways from a very young age. As discussed earlier in relation to the gut–brain axis (page 27), the food we eat has a huge impact on our mind. Furthermore, several studies talk about a link between depression and insulin resistance.[73, 74, 75, 76, 77] The exact mechanism is not known, but as this book shows, there are many causes for insulin resistance. An unbalanced gut microbiome is one of them. All these problems can affect our mind severely. A more recent study found that people suffering from insulin resistance reacted to stress with greater negative feelings than those with a healthy metabolism.[78] As mentioned before, the brain as one of our vital organs can suffer from insulin resistance like all the other organs too and so reversing insulin resistance would be the most important treatment measure.

Chapter 5

Problems with anxiety, depression and stress start early and then continue throughout life. They often escalate, causing many difficult situations later in life as other aspects of mental health, such as concentration and learning, may be affected. Depression has also been shown to increase our risk of dementia.[79] Too often we see how negativity and anxiety affect everyone around us, in our families, schools and workplaces. When we feel bad and pessimistic ourselves, and life seems difficult, we tend to take it out on the people closest to us, or around us. You can see this every day, everywhere, even in doctors' surgeries or the supermarket – people raging about meaningless issues, unable to hold a proper conversation; parents shouting at their children with no patience, or ignoring them completely; road rage putting others in danger. These are very important issues; – we should try to talk about the root causes more.

When battling with stress, anxiety or any mental health problem, food is always the factor to look at first; try making some dietary changes before taking any other measures. This is important; even the more serious mental illnesses, such as schizophrenia, have been linked to insulin resistance,[80] at least in some patients, and there is already evidence available of the effectiveness of a low-carbohydrate diet in managing the symptoms. So these are the steps to take for better mental health; as you can see, they overlap considerably with the steps to reduce insulin resistance:

- cut out sugar
- follow a wholefood, low-carbohydrate diet
- take appropriate supplements
- reduce caffeine intake
- exercise regularly
- spend time in nature
- try meditation and deep breathing
- try aromatherapy.

In addition to reducing sugar and carbohydrates, we need to remember the importance of good quality food, as discussed earlier, to ensure all important micronutrients are available for the proper functioning of the brain. We have looked at the important measures for restoring a good balance in the gut (page 99) and the need to ensure we are getting enough omega-3 fatty acids from our diet (page 95). All these form a good foundation to stress management or treatment of any mental illness, even when medication is needed. It is easier to manage stress and other mental health problems once dietary issues have been sorted. Nearly all of my patients tell me that after starting a low-carbohydrate, whole-food diet, all the things that had been causing them anger and irritation become unimportant. They generally feel calmer and more peaceful and find stressful situations in everyday life are no longer that bad. They feel much more positive and nothing gets them too angry. No more road-rage or temper tantrums!

In addition to foods, there are some supplements available specifically to help deal with stress and anxiety. The most important is vitamin D as deficiencies have been linked to both insulin resistance and mental problems such as depression.[81, 82] Omega-3 supplements are beneficial for those who don't eat fish.[83, 84, 85, 86, 87] EPA fatty acid in particular is a powerful antidepressive. Ashwagandha might also help, with studies to back up its possible effectiveness;[88] please find out more from a functional practitioner if interested. Green tea has also been found to help in managing stress and anxiety, possibly due to the polyphenols it contains.[89]

Be careful with coffee and tea as high intake can increase anxiety in some people.

Exercise has a very positive effect on our mind, as explained earlier (page 30). We all know this in principal, but we should try and get out into the fresh air regularly also. Walking in nature is an especially good stress management tool; it can lower our stress hormone levels very effectively, improve our mood and immunity, and lower our blood pressure[90, 91, 92] – definitely an extremely effective way of treating insulin resistance in addition to other measures. For this reason I have always found it important to go outdoors with my family regularly, to teach my children to enjoy nature from a very early age. In the past, nature has always been a very important part of our lives, but unfortunately today many people don't have enough time even to go out for a walk. However, even in a park if you live in an urban area, away from any woodland, it is possible to sit down or walk and enjoy the natural world around you.

Meditation, mindfulness and deep breathing have also been found to have a positive effect on our blood sugar levels[93, 94, 95] and are worth trying, even if only for a few minutes every day. Like other stress management measures, they also lower levels of the stress hormones cortisol and adrenaline and calm us down. In addition, like exercise, meditation can also release hormones like serotonin, oxytocin and dopamine, which improve our mood significantly and also have a positive impact on our concentration and memory.

Meditation can mean many different things. Walking in a quiet forest/woodland has a very meditative feeling to it, as does sitting comfortably in peace and quiet for a few moments on the edge of the bed before starting the daily routine. When meditating, we often not only notice our body and how we are feeling, but we also concentrate on our breathing. Deep breathing and noticing how we inhale and exhale go hand in hand with meditation and form the basis of meditation and relaxation. Deep breathing usually called 'belly breathing' or 'diaphragmatic breathing', is known to reduce stress levels and blood pressure and to help us sleep better. Relaxing, meditating and breathing might not sound like much, but because we know already how chronic stress affects us in so many ways – for example, by lowering our immunity – we know that even these simple measures will help improve our lives and bring additional benefits when reversing insulin resistance.

Relaxing, meditation and mindful breathing might not sound like much but these simple measures can lower stress and thereby improve immunity and help reverse insulin resistance

Essential oils might also help. Some people find, for example, that candles, bath salts and/or body oils containing certain essential oils are very soothing and there are studies available showing the benefits of aromatherapy in reducing stress and anxiety and improving sleep.[96, 97]

Sleep well

Good quality sleep is likewise very important for our health. The connection between insulin resistance and sleep disturbances was explained on page 24. There is no function in our body that is not affected by lack of sleep, but insomnia is unfortunately very common.

Reversing insulin resistance effectively, plus stress management measures, helps to improve sleep. Problems such as snoring and/or sleep apnoea improve dramatically when insulin resistance is reversed and the overall hormonal balance is restored. All this helps to balance our gut microbiome, improving the production of the sleep hormone melatonin.

In addition to reversing insulin resistance, it is important for us all to use some other good sleep hygiene measures in everyday life to make sure that we sleep well, as often as possible. This is to ensure there are no other disturbances ruining our sleep. According to studies, just one night of poor sleep can lower our insulin sensitivity.[98]

Chapter 5

Problems such as snoring and sleep apnoea improve dramatically when insulin resistance is reversed

One of the most important sleep hygiene measures is to try to make sure to turn off all electronic devices, including mobile phones and the TV, well before bedtime, to minimise the amount of artificial light, which is known to disturb our sleep. Just enjoy a good book instead before bed if you like reading. It has also been found to be beneficial to stick to a certain sleep routine, which means that we go to sleep more or less at the same time each night, and wake up at the same time every morning. For most of us, caffeine, as a stimulant, has an effect on our sleep, so if you experience any sleep problems, it might be a good idea to avoid any caffeine-containing drinks after early afternoon. Alcohol is another substance that has an effect. Although it makes us sleepy, the quality of sleep after drinking even small amounts of alcohol is often poor as alcohol prevents us from reaching the deep stages of sleep.

Exercising too late in the evening can also disturb your sleep but some people find that something more calming, such as yoga, stretching and/or meditating before bed can be very helpful. Also making sure that your bed is comfortable and the temperature in your bedroom is not too high helps in getting a good night's sleep.

Chapter 6

Special considerations

Possible problems with a low-carbohydrate diet

As ever, when starting a new lifestyle, there can be some side effects and this is true when starting a low-carbohydrate diet, particularly if you have been eating a lot of carbs and especially sugar in the past.

One of the main problems is that, as explained earlier, insulin causes our kidneys to retain sodium, which in the presence of insulin resistance and hyperinsulinaemia results in fluid retention and raised blood pressure. When our insulin levels drop when following a diet low in carbohydrates, our body starts to remove this excess sodium as well as excess fluids, often quickly. If those sodium levels, which affect levels of other minerals too, drop quickly, we end up with symptoms such as headaches, fatigue and weakness as a result. It is important therefore, not to forget to include salt in your diet. Eating a whole food diet and avoiding processed foods usually means that the diet does not contain a lot of sodium. This is why added salt is a good idea, to avoid the symptoms mentioned. There are many different opinions on the exact amount of salt we should eat. For example the NHS recommends no more than 1 teaspoon of salt a day,[1] but there are also worries about consuming inadequate amounts of sodium,[2, 3] which can be harmful, especially if your blood pressure is normal. If you experience any side effects when reversing insulin resistance, it is important to replace the lost sodium, so you can try adding small amount of salt into your food, or eat foods such as olives or pickles with added salt.

The most common side effect is to experience flu-like symptoms for a short while. You might feel slightly unwell for two to three days after starting the diet. The symptoms might include headache, dizziness, mild nausea, irritability and fatigue, or occasionally cramps. These symptoms usually settle quickly when your body adapts to your new lifestyle.

These side effects are almost always caused by loss of salts, including sodium in particular, but also potassium and magnesium. It is important to remember to drink enough fluids and, as I have said, add enough salt to your food to minimise these symptoms. Also, eating foods containing potassium, such as almonds, yoghurt, eggs, salmon and mushrooms, might help. If you experience any leg cramps, Epsom salts are a very good remedy for this; they are made of magnesium sulphate and can be absorbed through the skin so putting them in your bath or footbath can help muscles to relax.

Constipation is another side effect that some people experience at the start of this diet. Usually it is caused by dehydration so again, remember to drink enough and make sure you are getting enough salt. Eat plenty of vegetables to ensure you are also getting enough fibre. Some people have found a few spoonfuls of olive oil or coconut oil daily very helpful.

Heart palpitations might be present sometimes; these again are usually caused by dehydration and lack of salt. If a result of the change of diet, they are harmless and should pass, but if there are any concerns, consult your doctor.

By 'salt' of course we mainly mean salt that contains two minerals – sodium and chloride – both essential for the body. Regular table salt, however, is refined salt which often contains other substances too, for example anti-caking agents. Other salts, such as sea salt and Himalayan salt often contain traces of other minerals, such as potassium, zinc, magnesium and iron. They also contain slightly less sodium compared with regular table salt. For these reasons I consider these salts to be a better option.

Please note that if you have any medical conditions that you take medication for, especially type 1 or type 2 diabetes or high blood pressure, you will need to consult a knowledgeable doctor before starting this diet. This is because a low-carb diet will lower both your blood sugar and your blood pressure and your medication will need to be adapted very quickly. There are also many websites available, such as diabetes.co.uk, with plenty of information about low-carbohydrate eating and medication.

Addictions and food cravings

Craving carbohydrates is a real problem for many people. Very often even small amounts of bread or pasta in your food cause cravings: you end up craving more carb-filled food and before you know it, your new lifestyle has gone wrong. It is often easier to avoid starchy carbohydrates, such as bread, and especially sugar entirely rather than trying to eat them in moderation. Most of us have tried a calorie-restricted diet in the past and this is exactly why it is almost impossible to stay on these diets in the long term. The more carbs you eat, the more insulin you release and the more you crave those carbs. Blood sugar levels fluctuate too much.

Carbohydrates, and especially sugar, also trigger the brain reward centre, just like drugs. Sugar can be just as addictive and just as difficult to cut out.

When eating only small amounts of carbohydrate in the form of non-starchy vegetables, if you avoid sugar completely and include lots of healthy fats in your diet, any addiction and binge behaviour will stop and it will become a lot easier to stay on a healthy diet. A low-carb diet could help in treating other addictions too. Certainly, it does seem that once following this type of diet, any possible cravings not only for sugar but also alcohol, are not so powerful anymore.

What about calories?

Most of us are still concerned about calories when it comes to eating. However, losing weight and restoring health are all about reversing insulin resistance, not about counting calories. As ex-plained in Chapter 1, our metabolism is very complex and different foods have completely different effects on our hormones, hunger and metabolic health. Therefore, all calories are definitely not the same, but different foods have different metabolic effects, even when they have the same amount of calories.

This is the reason why our previous way of looking at calories when trying to control weight and prevent metabolic disease has not worked; indeed, it has actually made things worse. Focusing on calories alone has led to the consumption of highly processed low-calorie foods. We have not realised that this type of food has increased problems with inflammation, micronutrient deficiencies and unbalanced gut microbiome – and insulin resistance has got worse, not better.

Focusing on calories has in particular prevented us from seeing the especially important role of insulin and how excess carbohydrates have actually made us more hungry, with fluctuating blood sugar levels. As a consequence, we have also needed increasing numbers of snacks throughout the day, which has led to many of us eating much more than we need. It is best not to think about calories, but focus only on reversing insulin resistance. This will restore our hormonal balance and help us to lose excess weight.

Pregnancy and 'gestational diabetes'

Unfortunately, insulin resistance and hyperinsulinaemia can cause problems in pregnancy also. Insulin sensitivity usually decreases anyway during pregnancy because of hormonal changes and the need for extra glucose for the growing foetus. Normally this is overcome by a slight increase in insulin production by the pancreas, but in the presence of insulin resistance before pregnancy, the increasing insulin levels will cause additional problems during pregnancy, even leading to possible gestational diabetes. It seems that the severity of insulin resistance varies throughout pregnancy and seems to be at its peak towards the third trimester.[11] This would therefore be an extremely important issue to look at during pregnancy in women with any symptoms of insulin resistance before pregnancy. We know insulin resistance during pregnancy, and especially gestational diabetes, can have long-term effects not only on the metabolic health of the mother but also on the unborn child,[4] often manifesting in childhood.

It seems maternal insulin cannot easily cross the placenta,[5] but it has an important role in glucose metabolism between the mother and unborn baby, so it is very central in the proper functioning of the placenta. There seem to be only a very few studies looking into how the mother's insulin resistance affects the pregnancy, but we know that hyperinsulinaemia affects the structure and the functioning of the placenta because of damage to the vulnerable placental cells, especially during the first trimester. This can even lead to miscarriages in early pregnancy.[6, 7] The higher the levels of insulin are, the more harmful it is for the placenta. Inflammation, oxidative stress and the associated mitochondrial dysfunctions explain this effect, although the exact mechanism is still unknown.

Too much glucose in the mother's bloodstream will cross the placenta, causing hyperinsulinaemia in the growing baby

Glucose does cross the placenta and if there is too much

glucose in the mother's bloodstream ('gestational diabetes'), the pancreas of the foetus releases increasing amounts of insulin which leads to hyperinsulinaemia of the foetus. This causes inflammation and changes in gene expression and increases the size of both the foetus and the placenta.[8, 9, 10] This in turn can cause abnormalities in the development of both, even stillbirth or the death of the baby shortly after birth, mostly caused by increasing oxygen demands which cannot be met, as well as lack of nutrients. Complications during the delivery are also more likely due to the larger size of the baby.

Children and teenagers

I wanted to include a few words about childhood and teenage obesity, and other health problems, because they are such huge issues in the world today and cause so many ill effects at such a precious age. I have a lot of experience – both personal and professional – of how effective the dietary measures for reversing insulin resistance explained in Chapter 5 can be in young people; this is absolutely the best treatment. I have seen many excellent examples of this. With young patients, simply cutting out sugar and excess refined carbohydrates, such as bread and cereals, and increasing the nutrient content of foods by eating real food and avoiding processed food, has had a massive impact on any health problem they had. They have lost excess weight very quickly and safely, without feeling hungry. I wish there was more awareness of insulin resistance when dealing with these problems because excess weight has such a big effect on young people's lives.

The quality of food is also so important when it comes to growing children. They need lots of good quality, natural fat and good quality protein, in addition to all the important micronutrients for all their body functions and development. When we keep this in mind, we can also help with many other common problems young people are facing, such as eczema, acne, abdominal symptoms and anxiety.

Of course, this is challenging when there is so much sugar and processed food around us. However, what I have found helpful is just explaining the metabolism and the effects of foods such as sugar on our body to the young person, or parents of a younger child, so that they learn about why some foods have a damaging effect.

Insulin resistance and the menopause

Symptoms of menopause start to affect women around the age of 45-55 as the levels of the hormones oestrogen, progesterone and testosterone start to change. This causes changes in the menstrual cycle and often mood swings as well as other difficult symptoms such as hot flushes and night sweats. Often these symptoms start months, or even years, before the woman's periods stop. These changes in hormone levels increase the risk of insulin resistance, or they can make existing insulin resistance worse,[12] so, in the presence of insulin resistance, it can be very difficult to manage the symptoms of menopause.

The symptoms of insulin-induced 'oestrogen dominance' and menopause are very difficult to tell apart but both can be relieved with a low-carb diet

As we have learned in Chapter 4, insulin resistance has a major effect on our whole hormonal balance. One of the consequences is a condition called 'oestrogen dominance', where there are high levels of oestrogen in the body compared with progesterone levels (page 51). There are many symptoms of this imbalance, including tiredness, problems with periods, mood swings and sleep disturbances – very similar symptoms to the menopause. It is therefore very difficult sometimes to know the cause of symptoms in women who are approaching menopause.

For women going through the menopause, when the body

is already trying to manage an imbalance of sex hormones, the problems caused by underlying insulin resistance can be severe. When oestrogen levels fall after the menopause, the inflammation caused by underlying insulin resistance may rapidly increase, which again increases the risk of complications even further.

It would be important for all women going through the menopause to manage their symptoms with those measures I have described throughout this book. This would reduce the risk of insulin problems caused by the hormonal changes in menopause and/or treat underlying insulin resistance, making menopause easier.

Chapter 7

How do I eat to reverse insulin resistance?

Sample meals

The purpose of the recipes in this chapter is to share ideas of different meals you can have when reversing insulin resistance. This diet is not at all difficult to follow; it is only a question of preparing good homemade, ordinary, real food for the whole family, but without starch or sugar.

The easiest way to start in my opinion is to eat the same types of meal you normally do, but swap the starchy foods you have had in the past with a variety of vegetables. For example, instead of potatoes, choose steamed broccoli or sliced cabbage; instead of a sandwich, prepare a salad or a soup. Be bold enough to try many different, new vegetables you might not have considered in the past. Roast them in the oven, boil, steam, or stirfry them, and you will soon notice that they actually taste a lot better than potatoes or pasta. Don't forget to try herbs too. Then enjoy good protein with your veggies – that could be fish, meat, eggs, cheese or a vegetarian option, such as tofu, and natural fat, such as extra-virgin olive oil.

If you like to have a breakfast, then coffee with some cream is often a good choice. Small amounts of berries and perhaps a few nuts and seeds with yoghurt or crème fraîche are great, or you can have eggs in some form. Green smoothies are also a very good choice as long as they are mostly vegetable-based and you are careful with the amount of fruit.

Remember to drink plenty of water during the day. I also like herbal teas. Green tea, peppermint and nettle are my favourites, but try a good variety. Ordinary coffee and tea are absolutely fine as long as you don't add any sugar or sweetener and are careful with milk because it contains the sugar lactose.

Cost

Many people worry about the cost of a healthy diet. We have noticed that it is easy to stay within our budget because we eat less often than before and never buy anything extra, such as cereals, crisps, sugary yoghurts or puddings. We invest in large amounts of good seasonal veg, often directly from the market or small producers, which is always cheaper, and then you know where your food comes from, which is important. Many supermarkets do have good and affordable selections also. For example, cabbage is cheap and very nutritious; pumpkins are also lovely when in season (see Pumpkin soup below – page 121). We also eat lots of eggs in different forms. Cheaper cuts of meat (the delicious fattier cuts) and liver are also usually lower in price, as is locally-caught fish if available in your area.

Please note that if you have any sensitivity to specific foods – for example, a milk-protein or nut allergy – you should of course follow your doctor's recommendations.

Chapter 7

Soups

Chicken-coconut soup

For 4 people

- 500 ml chicken stock
- 1 can coconut milk (400 ml)
- 2 tbsp Thai green curry paste
- small piece (approx. 4 cm) fresh ginger, sliced
- 200 g mushrooms
- 2 tbsp lime or lemon juice
- 2 tbsp (or according to taste) soya sauce
- 2 red chillies, cut into thin slices (optional)
- 1 handful fresh Thai basil
- 1 handful fresh coriander
- 4 spring onions, chopped
- 350-400 g cooked chicken, either leftovers from a roast, or 2 chicken breasts, sliced and stir fried until cooked through

> **Bring the chicken stock and coconut milk to the boil.**
> **Add the curry paste, ginger, mushrooms and lime/lemon juice and, according to your preference, the soya sauce and chillies.**
> **Simmer for 5 minutes.**
> **Add the chicken, spring onions and fresh chopped herbs.**

Leek and broccoli soup

For 4 people

- 1 large leek (or 2-3 small ones)
- 1 large head broccoli
- 1 clove garlic, chopped
- 250 g cream cheese
- small knob of butter
- 1 handful fresh basil, chopped
- salt
- black pepper

Cut the leek and broccoli core into slices.

In a saucepan, cook them in a small amount of water until just soft.

Add the broccoli florets and chopped garlic and simmer until the florets are tender.

Add the cream cheese and butter, season with salt and black pepper and add the fresh basil.

With a hand blender, blend until smooth, adding more water if needed.

If you like, you can add some cream.

Reheat carefully if needed and serve the soup hot.

Chapter 7

Pumpkin soup

For 4 people

- 800 g pumpkin, chopped
- half an apple, chopped
- olive oil
- 1-2 cloves garlic, grated
- 2-cm piece fresh ginger, grated
- 500 ml chicken stock
- 100-200 ml coconut cream
- 1 pinch of dried chilli flakes

Sauté the pumpkin and apple in olive oil for a short while until slightly softened.
Add the garlic, ginger and then the chicken stock and simmer until the pumpkin is soft.
Blend the soup with a hand blender.
Add the coconut cream, stir well and decorate with some dried chilli flakes.

Fish-coconut soup

For 4 people

- 1 onion, chopped
- 2 cloves garlic, grated
- 4-5 cm piece fresh ginger, grated
- 1 red chilli peper, sliced
- 700 ml fish stock (or water)
- 1 courgette, cut into chunks
- 2 carrots, sliced
- 1 yellow pepper, sliced
- 1 can coconut milk (400 ml)
- 400 g cod fillets (or another white fish), cut into large chunks
- 1 tbsp tomato purée
- juice from half a lime
- salt
- black pepper
- 1 handful fresh parsley or coriander, chopped

Sauté the onion, garlic, ginger and chilli in a large sauce pan for 2 minutes.
Add the stock or water, courgette, carrots and pepper; bring to the boil and simmer for 5 minutes.
Add the coconut milk, fish and the tomato purée and stir carefully.
Bring to the boil, cover and simmer for 3-4 minutes until the fish is cooked through.
Add the lime juice and season with salt and pepper.
Garnish with the fresh herbs.

Chapter 7

Spinach soup

For 4 people

- olive oil
- 1 onion, chopped
- 250 g fresh baby spinach
- 600 ml chicken or vegetable stock
- 200-250 g cream cheese or soft goats' cheese
- 2 cloves garlic, chopped or grated
- 1 small handful fresh parsley or thyme, chopped
- salt
- black pepper

Sauté the onion in olive oil in a saucepan for 1-2 minutes until it is soft.
Mix in the spinach and stir for another 1-2 minutes.
Then add the stock and bring to the boil.
Add the garlic and herbs and blend until smooth using a hand blender.
Stir in the cheese, and blend again until smooth.
Season with salt and pepper according to your taste.

Lunches

Homemade quiche

For 6-8 people

You can try any topping. We like the classic bacon and cheese so this is what I describe here.

For the base:
- 100 g butter (soft, room temperature)
- 2 eggs
- 300 ml ground almonds

Pre-heat the oven to 180°C.
Mix all the ingredients together with your fingers and then pat the mix carefully into the bottom of a buttered quiche dish.
Cook in the oven for 15 minutes and then allow to cool.

For the topping:
- 6 rashers bacon
- 1 onion
- 3 eggs
- 200 ml cream
- 200 g grated cheese, such as gruyere or cheddar
- salt
- black pepper

Cut the bacon and onion into cubes and gently sauté in a pan, in butter or olive oil.
In a bowl, whisk the eggs and mix in the cream carefully.
Pour the mixture on to the base, add the bacon and onion, and sprinkle with the grated cheese.
Return to the oven for another 30-40 minutes, until cooked through and golden brown.

Chapter 7

Kale-onion-goats' cheese pie

For 6 people

For the base:
- 300 ml cauliflower and broccoli, cooked
- 3 eggs
- 200 ml almond flour (or ground almond)
- 2 tsp psyllium husk
- 1 tsp salt

> Pre-heat the oven to 180°C.
> Mash the cooked cauliflower and broccoli with a fork or blender.
> Mix all the ingredients in a bowl and spread into a pie dish which has been greased with olive oil first.
> Place the dish in the oven for 15 minutes.

Topping:
- 3-4 handfuls kale
- 3-4 spring onions
- 50 g goats' cheese
- 200 ml coconut cream
- 3 eggs
- 300 ml grated cheese
- salt
- black pepper
- white pepper

> Chop the kale into small pieces and slice the spring onions.
> Chop the goats' cheese into small pieces.
> Mix the kale, spring onions and goats' cheese together and spoon over the pre-cooked base.
> Whisk the eggs, add the cream and mix.
> Add the grated cheese, salt and pepper, and pour over the filling.
> Return the dish to the oven for 20-25 minutes, until golden brown on top.

Vegetable frittata

For 4-6 people

- 2 tbsp olive oil
- 100 g tenderstem broccoli, cut into smaller pieces
- 2 red peppers, cut into thin slices
- 6 large eggs
- 50 ml double cream
- salt
- black pepper
- 100 g feta cheese, crumbled

Pre-heat the oven to 180°C.
Heat approx 2 tbsp of olive oil in a frying pan.
Add the broccoli and peppers and stir-fry for about 5 minutes, until the vegetables have softened.
Transfer them to an oven-proof dish that you have greased with olive oil.
Whisk the eggs in a jug, mix in the cream and season with salt and pepper.
Add the egg mix to the oven-proof dish and then the crumbled feta cheese.
Place the dish in the oven for 10 minutes or until the feta cheese is slightly golden brown on the top.
Serve with a green salad.

Chapter 7

Goats' cheese and bacon salad

For 2 people

- 100 g goats' cheese, cut into 1 cm thick slices
- 4 rashers thin-cut streaky bacon
- 2 large handfuls lettuce or salad leaves of your choice, for example rocket
- 10 cherry tomatoes
- 50 g walnuts

For the dressing:
- 3 tbsp olive oil
- 1 tbsp balsamic vinegar
- 1 tsp honey
- 1 small red pepper, very finely chopped
- salt
- black pepper

Pre-heat the oven to 180°C.
Arrange baking paper in an oven-proof dish.
Place the goats' cheese slices in the dish and bake in the oven until crispy and golden on top.
Fry the bacon in a frying pan until crispy.
Place the lettuce or salad leaves in a salad bowl and add the cherry tomatoes on top.
Cut the fried bacon into pieces and place on top of the salad, and then add the goats' cheese slices on top of that.
Sprinkle with the walnuts.
Mix all the dressing ingredients together and season with salt and black pepper, then drizzle over the salad.

Greek salad

For 4 people

- 100 g Kalamata olives (or more if you like)
- 4 tomatoes, cut into large chunks
- half a cucumber, halved lengthwise and then cut into thick slices
- 1 red onion, cut in half and then thinly sliced
- 1 green pepper, sliced
- 3-4 tbsp olive oil
- 1-2 tbsp red wine vinegar
- 200 g feta cheese
- ½ tbsp dried oregano
- some fresh mint leaves

Place all the vegetables in a large salad dish, including the olives.
Pour on the olive oil and red wine vinegar and toss.
Add the feta cheese on top.
Sprinkle the dried oregano over the top and garnish with some fresh mint leaves.

Chapter 7

Smoked mackerel salad

For 4 people

- 200 g cherry tomatoes, halved
- 2 handfuls salad leaves of your choice
- 250 g pack ready-cooked puy lentils (optional)
- 1 handful fresh chives, chopped
- 150 g smoked mackerel, skinned, broken into bite-size chunks
- juice of ½ lemon
- olive oil

> **Put the tomatoes, salad leaves and lentils (if using) into a salad bowl and mix carefully.**
> **Add the chives and the mackerel.**
> **Squeeze on the lemon juice, drizzle with olive oil, gently toss and serve.**
>
> *Please note that lentils contain more carbohydrates than vegetables; in the packet used in this recipe, there are just over 11 g of carbohydrates per person.*

Baked salmon and spinach

For 4 people

- 4 fillets salmon
- olive oil
- salt
- black pepper
- 100 ml sour cream
- 50 g parmesan cheese, grated
- 400 g fresh baby spinach leaves

Pre-heat the oven to 200°C.
Place the salmon fillets in an oven-proof dish you have greased with olive oil, skin-side down and season with salt and black pepper.
Mix the sour cream and parmesan, and spread over the salmon fillets.
Bake for 15-20 minutes, until the salmon is cooked through.
Sauté the spinach in a pan, in a small amount of olive oil, or butter, for 2 minutes and serve with the salmon fillets.

Chapter 7

Courgette and smoked fish cakes

Makes 16-18 small cakes

- 1 courgette (approx 300 g), coarsely grated
- 300 g cooked smoked fish without the skin and bones, flaked with a fork – you can use any fish in this recipe
- 150 g grated cheese, such as cheddar
- 2 eggs
- 1 tbsp grated lemon zest
- 1 tsp psyllium husk (optional)
- salt
- black pepper

For the dill-lemon sauce:
- 150 g crème fraîche or sour cream
- 2 tbsp lemon juice
- 2 tbsp chopped fresh dill

> Mix all the sauce ingredients together and let the sauce set in the fridge for a while.
> Mix together all the fish cake ingredients and form small burger-shaped cakes with your fingers.
> Fry them on both sides until golden brown.
> Serve the warm fish cakes with the cold sauce.

Mediterranean eggs

For 4 people

- 3-4 tbsp olive oil
- 2 onion, chopped
- 1 red pepper, finely chopped
- 2 large tomatoes, chopped
- 2 cloves garlic, finely sliced or chopped
- salt
- black pepper
- paprika
- 4 eggs
- 1 small handful fresh coriander, chopped

Heat the olive oil in a large frying pan or skillet with a lid.
Fry the onion and pepper for about 5 minutes, until they have softened.
Add the tomatoes and garlic and season with salt, pepper and a sprinkling of paprika.
Stir and simmer for 10 minutes until the juices have been cooked off.
Make 4 small holes/dips in the mixture (or more if using more eggs) with the back of a wooden spoon and crack the eggs into them.
Cover the skillet and cook on a low heat for another 5-6 minutes until the eggs are cooked to your liking; he yolks should still be runny.
Scatter with chopped coriander and serve immediately.

Easy sauerkraut

Makes enough for a 1-1.5-litre jar

- 1 whole white cabbage (approx 1-1.5 kg)
- 20 g sea salt (or pink Himalayan rock salt) per kilo

Grate the cabbage, or cut it into very thin slices.
Place it in a large bowl, add the salt and massage together for a few minutes, until the cabbage starts to break.
Transfer the cabbage and salt to a large, sterilised, air-tight glass jar (with a wide opening), pressing it down tightly.
Pour in any juices left in the bowl.
Close the jar lid and leave the jar at room temperature.
Each day open the lid to release the gas forming as a result of fermentation.
The sauerkraut should be ready to eat in a week, but you can keep it longer to mature.

Dinners

Spaghetti squash with garlic mushrooms

For 2-4 people

For the 'spaghetti':
- 1 spaghetti squash
- olive oil
- salt
- black pepper

> Pre-heat the oven to 180-200°C.
> Cut the squash in half lengthwise and scoop out the seeds.
> Drizzle the cut side with some olive oil and season with salt and black pepper.
> Place the squash in an oven-proof dish lined with baking paper, cut side down and prick a few holes in it with a fork.
> Roast for 30-40 minutes, until it is slightly browned; the roasting time depends on the size of the squash.
> Remove from the oven, turn it over and let it cool a little until it is cool enough to handle, then use a fork to scrape and fluff the strands from the squash. They look like spaghetti.

For the garlic mushrooms:
- 2 tbsp olive oil
- 200 g button mushrooms, cut in half
- 2 cloves garlic, grated
- 100 g parmesan cheese, grated
- small handful fresh parsley, chopped
- salt
- black pepper

Chapter 7

> Heat the olive oil in a pan.
> Add the mushrooms and garlic and fry until the mushrooms are golden brown, which will take 6-7 minutes.
> Add the spaghetti squash strands, stir carefully and sauté for a further minute.
> Sprinkle with grated parmesan cheese and season with salt and black pepper.
> Sprinkle with the freshly chopped parsley.

You can also serve the squash with your favourite spaghetti sauce, such as the Bolognese sauce.

Greek meatballs and tzatziki sauce

For 6 people

For the meatballs:
- 500 g beef mince
- 500 g lamb mince
- 1 onion, finely chopped
- 3 cloves garlic, grated
- 2 eggs
- small handful fresh mint leaves, chopped
- zest of 1 lemon, grated
- 2 tsp ground coriander
- 2 tsp dried oregano
- 2 tsp ground cumin
- salt
- black pepper
- olive oil

Mix together all the ingredients apart from the olive oil.
To get the level of spices to your liking, you can fry a small amount of meat mixture for tasting and then adjust the spices if needed.
Using your fingers, form balls from the meat mixture and set aside.
Heat 2-3 tablespoons of olive oil in a large frying pan and fry the meatballs in batches until cooked through and golden brown.
Alternatively, you can bake the meatballs in the oven (200°C) in an oven-proof dish lined with baking paper; drizzle some olive oil over the meatballs and bake them in the oven for 20-30 minutes, turning them over halfway through.
Serve the meatballs with the tzatziki sauce (next) and a Greek salad (page 128).

Chapter 7

For the tzatziki sauce

- 1 small cucumber, grated or finely chopped
- 1 tsp salt
- 500 g thick Greek yoghurt
- small handful fresh dill, finely chopped
- few leaves fresh mint, finely chopped
- 1-2 cloves garlic, grated
- 1 tbsp lemon juice
- 1 tbsp olive oil
- salt
- black pepper

> Mix the grated cucumber with 1 tsp salt and place in a sieve/colander to drain for 30 minutes.
> Squeeze the water out of the cucumber and transfer to a bowl.
> Add the yoghurt, herbs, garlic, lemon juice and olive oil.
> Mix well and season with salt and black pepper.

Pan-fried liver with sage and cream sauce

For 4 people

For the sage and cream sauce:
- small knob of butter
- 1 small onion, finely chopped
- small handful fresh sage, finely chopped
- 100 ml white wine
- 200 ml cream
- 1 tsp Dijon-mustard
- salt
- black pepper

Sauté the onion in a small amount of butter, for a few minutes.
Add the sage, stir and then add the wine.
Bring to the boil and let the wine reduce until half of it is left.
Add the cream and mustard, stir and season with salt and pepper.
Simmer for 10 minutes.
Meanwhile prepare the liver.

For the pan-fried liver
- 400-450 lambs' or calves' liver, sliced
- small knob of butter
- salt
- black pepper

Melt the butter in a large frying pan.
Fry the liver slices for 2-3 minutes per side, until cooked, but still slightly pink in the middle; be careful not to over-cook.
Season with salt and black pepper and serve with the sage and cream sauce.

Cod casserole with mushrooms

For 6 people

- 600-700 g fillets of cod, or any other white fish
- 100 g butter
- 400 g mushrooms, cut in half, or wedges if they are large
- small knob of butter
- small handful fresh parsley, chopped
- 400 ml double cream
- 2 tbsp Dijon mustard
- 150 g grated cheese
- salt
- black pepper

> Pre-heat the oven to 180°C.
> Place the fish fillets into an oven-proof dish you have greased well with olive oil; season with salt and black pepper.
> Melt the butter in a pan, add the mushrooms and cook until they have softened, which takes about 5 minutes.
> Season with salt and black pepper, and sprinkle with chopped fresh parsley.
> Pour in the cream, add the mustard, mix well and simmer for 6-8 minutes until the cream has reduced slightly.
> Pour the mushroom sauce over the fish and sprinkle with grated cheese.
> Bake in the oven for 25-30 minutes, until the fish fillets are cooked through.
> Serve with steamed broccoli or a green salad on the side.

Tuna bake

For 4 people

- small knob of butter
- 1 onion, chopped finely
- 1 green bell pepper, chopped finely
- 1 yellow bell pepper, chopped finely
- 3 tins tuna (about 400-450 g), in spring water or brine
- 200 ml sour cream
- 100 g parmesan cheese, grated
- salt
- black pepper

Pre-heat the oven to 200°C.
Melt the butter in a large pan and cook the onion and peppers until slightly softened.
Season with salt and pepper.
In a bowl, mix the tuna, sour cream and parmesan cheese and then transfer them to an oven-proof dish you have greased well with some olive oil.
Add the vegetables and stir carefully.
Bake in the oven for 15-20 minutes until golden brown on top.
Serve with a green salad.

Chapter 7

One-pan chicken and vegetables

For 4 people

- olive oil
- 4 boneless chicken breasts, cut into bite-size pieces
- 2 courgettes, cut in half lengthwise and then sliced
- 2 red peppers, cut into slices
- 1 red onion, cut into slices
- 1 broccoli, cut into florets
- 4 cloves garlic, grated
- juice of 1 lemon
- salt
- black pepper
- handful fresh parsley, chopped
- handful fresh coriander, chopped

Pre-heat the oven to 180 °C.
Mix together the raw chicken pieces and all the vegetables in a large oven pan, spread in one layer, and season with the spices.
Add the lemon juice and a good drizzle of olive oil, then carefully mix everything together.
Bake in the oven for about 20 minutes, until the chicken is cooked through.
Garnish with the fresh herbs.

Shepherd's pie with cauliflower

For 4 people

For the cauliflower mash:
- 2 cauliflowers (approx 600-700 g), broken into florets
- ½ leek, cut into slices
- 100 ml crème fraîche or sour cream
- small knob of butter
- 100 g cheddar cheese, grated
- salt
- black pepper

For the filling:
- knob of butter
- olive oil
- 2 onions, finely chopped
- 800 g lamb or beef mince
- 3-4 cloves garlic, finely chopped or grated
- 2 tbsp tomato purée
- 400 ml chicken or beef stock
- sprinkle dried thyme
- sprinkle dried basil
- salt
- black pepper

Pre-heat the oven to 180°C.
To make the filling first, heat 2-3 tablespoons of olive oil in a pan, with a small knob of butter.
Add the onions and sauté for 4-5 minutes until they are soft.
Add the mince and continue cooking until it is cooked through.
Add the garlic and tomato purée and mix well.
Then add the stock and the herbs, bring to boil and simmer for 20 minutes until the stock has reduced.
Season with salt and black pepper.

Chapter 7

While the filling is cooking, prepare the mash by steaming the cauliflower and leeks for 6-7 minutes until they are soft; alternatively you can cook them in a small amount of boiling water.

Mash them with a potato masher, then add the crème fraîche, half of the cheese and butter and mix well.

Season with salt and black pepper.

Transfer the mince into an oven-proof dish.

Cover with the cauliflower mixture and sprinkle the rest of the grated cheese on top.

Cook in the oven for 20-25 minutes, until golden brown.

Chilli con carne

For 4 people

- olive oil
- 500 g beef mince
- 1 onion, finely chopped
- 1 red pepper, finely chopped
- 1 yellow pepper, finely chopped
- 2-3 cloves garlic, finely chopped, or grated
- 400 g can chopped tomatoes
- 2 tbsp tomato purée
- 1-2 tsp chilli powder
- 2 tsp paprika
- 1 tsp ground cumin
- salt
- black pepper
- sour cream and grated cheddar cheese for serving

Heat a drizzle of olive oil in a pan.
Add the mince and cook until it is brown.
When the meat is nearly cooked, add the onion and peppers and continue cooking for another 5 minutes. Add the garlic, tomatoes, tomato purée and all the spices, including salt and pepper, according to your taste.
Simmer for 15-20 minutes.
Serve with grated cheese and a spoonful of sour cream on top as well as a green salad.

Chapter 7

Smoked haddock gratin

For 4 people

- olive oil or butter
- 500 g baby spinach leaves
- 10-12 cherry tomatoes
- 2 fillets smoked haddock
- 2 large fillets unsmoked haddock, skinned and cut into 4 portions
- salt
- black pepper

For the topping:
- 200 ml sour cream
- juice of half a lemon
- 100 g grated cheddar cheese
- small handful fresh chives, finely chopped

Pre-heat the oven to 180°C.
Scatter the spinach leaves evenly over the base of an oven-proof dish you have greased well with olive oil or melted butter.
Place the haddock fillets on top of the spinach together with the tomatoes.
Mix all the ingredients for the topping in a small bowl and season with pepper and a little salt.
Spread the mixture over the fish and spinach, and bake for 30 minutes until bubbling and golden.
Serve with roasted mixed vegetables.

Oven-roasted salmon with garlic

For 4 people

- 1 large salmon fillet (approx 600-700 g)
- 150 g tenderstem broccoli, cut in half lengthwise
- 1 small fennel, sliced
- 1 small courgette, cut into quarters lengthwise and then finger-length pieces
- 10-12 cherry tomatoes
- 100 g green beans
- olive oil
- salt
- black pepper

For the creamy sauce (optional):
- 200 g sour cream
- 1 tsp Dijon mustard
- small handful chives, chopped
- 1 tbsp lemon juice

Pre-heat the oven to 180°C.
Place the salmon fillet on an oven tray lined with baking paper, skin side down. Drizzle with olive oil.
In a bowl, mix all the vegetables together, drizzle with some olive oil and spread around the salmon.
Season the salmon and vegetables with salt and black pepper.
Cook in the oven for 20-30 minutes, until the salmon is cooked through.
Mix all the sauce ingredients in a bowl and serve with the salmon and the vegetables.

Chapter 7

Pork and pepper stew with cauliflower rice

For 4 people

- olive oil
- 500 g pork tenderloin or medallion steaks, cut into cubes
- 2 onions, sliced
- 2 red peppers, cut into bite size pieces
- 600ml chicken stock
- 2 tbsp tomato purée
- 200 g mushrooms, cut in half
- 2 cloves garlic, finely chopped or grated
- 2 tsp smoked paprika
- black pepper
- salt
- handful of fresh parsley, chopped

Heat 2-3 tbsp of olive oil in a pan and fry the pork until browned, then set aside.
Fry the onion and peppers.
Add the stock, tomato purée, mushrooms, garlic and the pork, cover the pan with a lid and simmer for 20-30 minutes, or until the pork is tender.
Season with salt, pepper and smoked paprika, according to your taste.
Scatter with the parsley and serve with cauliflower rice.

For the cauliflower rice:

- 1 cauliflower, broken into florets
- olive oil
- small knob of butter
- salt
- black pepper

Put the cauliflower into a food processor and quickly pulse a few times until it is broken down into coarse crumbles.
Heat a drizzle of olive oil in a pan, then fry the cauliflower quickly on high heat for 3-4 minutes, until it is light brown.
Serve immediately as a side dish.

Grilled cod with red salsa and tenderstem broccoli

For 4 people

- olive oil
- ½ red onion, finely chopped
- 2 cloves garlic, grated
- 400 g (1 tin) chopped tomatoes
- 1 pinch chilli flakes
- salt
- black pepper
- 2 large skinless cod loins, cut in half, or 4 smaller fillets
- 200 g tenderstem broccoli
- juice of ½ lime
- small handful fresh coriander, chopped

Heat a drizzle of olive oil in a pan.
Add the red onion and garlic and sauté for 2 minutes until slightly softened.
Add the tomatoes, season with salt, pepper and a pinch of chilli flakes and then simmer for 15 minutes until the salsa mix is thicker.
Add the lime and sprinkle with the coriander.
Meanwhile, place the cod in an oven-proof dish, season well with salt and pepper and grill for 5-6 minutes, until cooked through.
Steam the broccoli until soft and serve with the cod and salsa.

Chapter 7

Baked portobello mushrooms with mozzarella, peppers and pesto

For 2-3 people

- 4-6 portobello mushrooms

For the filling:
- 300 g fresh mozzarella (2 x 150 g mozzarella balls)
- 1 red pepper, cut in half lengthwise, seeds and the top removed
- 100 ml black olives, stoned and sliced
- salt
- black pepper

For the marinade:
- 100 ml olive oil
- 2 tbsp balsamic vinegar

For the pesto:
- large handful of fresh chopped herbs: basil, parsley and thyme
- 2 cloves garlic, grated
- 100 ml olive oil
- 75 g pine nuts
- 100 ml grated parmesan cheese
- salt
- black pepper

Clean the mushrooms, brushing off any dirt.
Remove the stalks and chop them into very small cubes.
Brush the tops of the mushrooms with a small amount of olive oil, then place them upside down in a large oven-proof pan or oven tray, lined with baking paper.
Mix the olive oil and balsamic vinegar to make a marinade, spoon some of it inside the mushrooms and let them sit for half an hour. Save the rest of the marinade.
Grill the pepper halves in the oven until the skins have darkened.

Set them aside in a dish, cover with cling-film (being careful not to let the cling-film touch the pepper halves) and then, after 10 minutes, you should be able to remove the skins from the pepper halves.

Chop the peppers into very small cubes.

Prepare the pesto by mixing all the chopped herbs, garlic, olive oil and pine nuts and blend until smooth. Then add the parmesan and season with salt and pepper.

Chop the mozzarella into very small cubes.

Mix in a bowl with the mushroom stalk cubes and pepper cubes, the olives and as much pesto as you like. Season with salt and black pepper.

Spoon the filling into the portobello mushrooms, then pour over the rest of the marinade.

Bake in the oven (180°C) for 10 minutes until the cheese has melted. Garnish with some chopped fresh herbs.

This is a very tasty dish to have as a light lunch or dinner, or a lovely side dish.

Stuffed peppers with beef filling

For 4 people

- 4 large bell peppers
- olive oil
- 1 red onion, finely chopped
- 500 g beef mince
- salt
- pepper
- 2 cloves garlic, grated
- 400 g tomato passata
- sprinkle dried mixed herbs
- 100 g sour cream
- 4 large bell peppers
- 100 g grated cheese

Pre-heat the oven to 180°C.
Heat 2-3 tbsp of olive oil in a pan.
Add the onion, sauté for a few minutes, and then add the mince and cook until brown.
Season with salt and black pepper.
Add the garlic, tomato passata and a pinch of mixed herbs.
Simmer for 20 minutes.
Add the sour cream and mix well.
Cut the peppers in half, lengthwise, remove the seeds and place them, cut-side up, in a large oven-proof dish you have greased well with olive oil.
Spoon the filling into the peppers and sprinkle with the grated cheese.
Cook in the oven for 30-40 minutes.
Let the peppers set for 10-15 minutes before serving.
Serve with a green salad.

Fish curry

For 4-6 people

- small knob of butter or ghee
- 2 onions, sliced
- 3-4 cloves garlic, grated
- 2-3 cm piece fresh ginger, grated
- 1 green chilli sliced
- 1 tsp mustard seeds
- 2 tsp turmeric
- 2 tsp chilli powder
- 18-20 curry leaves
- 400 ml (1 tin) coconut milk
- 400 ml (1 tin) chopped tomatoes
- 600–700 g fish fillets, bones removed and chopped into bite-size pieces
- salt
- black pepper
- small handful of fresh coriander, chopped

Heat a small knob of butter or ghee in a pan.
Sauté the onion slices in the oil for a few minutes.
Add the garlic, ginger, chilli, spices and curry leaves.
Cook for a further few minutes.
Add the coconut milk and tomatoes.
Bring to the boil, cover the pan and simmer for 10-15 minutes.
Check the spices and add more if needed.
Add the fish pieces carefully to the sauce and simmer for 3-5 minutes, until the fish is cooked through.
Top with the fresh coriander.
Serve with cauliflower rice (see page 147).

Chapter 7

Beef goulash and celeriac mash

For 6 people

- olive oil and/or small knob of butter
- 1 kg braising steak, cut into bite-size chunks
- 3 onions cut into wedges
- 400 g (1 tin) chopped tomatoes
- 2 tbsp tomato purée
- 3 cloves garlic, chopped
- 1 tbsp paprika
- 2 tbsp hot smoked paprika
- 500 ml beef or chicken stock
- 1 green pepper, cut into bite-size cubes
- 1 red pepper, cut into bite-size cubes
- 1 yellow/orange pepper, cut into bite-size cubes
- salt
- black pepper

Pre-heat the oven to 150°C.
Heat a drizzle of olive oil and/or a knob of butter in an oven-proof pan or casserole dish.
Add the beef and stir-fry until browned all over.
Add the onions and for cook for 5 minutes until they soften.
Add the tomatoes, tomato purée, garlic, spices and stock.
Bring to the boil, cover and transfer the dish to the oven for 2 hours or until the meat is tender.
Add the peppers carefully to the dish and cook for a further hour.
Serve with celeriac mash.

For the celeriac mash (For 2-3 people)
- 1 whole celeriac (800 g) peeled and chopped into small cubes
- small knob of butter
- salt

Cook the celeriac in a small amount of water for 10 minutes until soft.
Drain and blend until smooth.
Add the butter and season with salt.

Aubergine parmigiana

For 4 people

- 2 aubergines, sliced thinly
- olive oil
- 100 g ricotta cheese
- 100 g mozzarella cheese, sliced
- 100 g parmesan cheese, grated
- salt
- black pepper

For the sauce:
- 1 red onion, finely chopped
- 3 cloves garlic, grated
- 2 tins (800 g) chopped tomatoes
- 100 ml red wine
- dried oregano
- small handful fresh basil

Pre-heat the oven to 200°C.
Brush the aubergine slices with olive oil on both sides.
Heat a frying pan and cook the slices, in batches, for 2 minutes per side, until they are slightly browned, then set them aside.
To prepare the sauce, add some olive oil to the pan and sauté the onion until soft.
Add the garlic, tomatoes, wine, oregano and basil.
Bring to the boil and simmer for 10-15 minutes, until the sauce thickens.
Grease an oven-proof dish with olive oil.
Spread a little sauce over the bottom of the dish, then add a layer of aubergine slices and spread another layer of the sauce on top of that.
Spread half of the ricotta cheese on top and sprinkle with parmesan cheese, salt and pepper.
Repeat the layers until the aubergine slices have all been used.
Add the mozzarella slices on the top and sprinkle with parmesan cheese.
Bake in the oven for 25 minutes, until golden brown.
Serve with a green salad.

Appendix

Low-, medium- and high-carbohydrate foods

Foods low in carbohydrate

These foods contain around 5 grams (g) of carbohydrate per 100 g, so they can be eaten freely when following a diet low in carbohydrates:

- **Most vegetables that grow above ground** – that is, different kinds of cabbages including Brussels sprouts and kale, broccoli, asparagus, avocado, cauliflower, mushrooms, cucumber, tomatoes, leafy greens, including spinach, olives, peppers.
- **Berries** – raspberries, blackberries, strawberries
- **Coconut**
- **Some other nuts and seeds** – macadamia nuts, Brazil nuts, pecans, hemp seeds
- **Some dairy products** – cheese, cream, sour cream, ricotta
- **Meat and poultry**
- **Eggs**
- **Fish and seafood**
- **Natural fat** – lard, ghee, coconut oil, cold-pressed extra-virgin olive oil
- **Fermented soy** – tofu, tempeh

Foods that contain a medium amount of carbohydrate

These foods contain more carbohydrate, usually between 7 and 13 g per 100 g, and so should only be eaten in moderation by people who suffer from insulin resistance. Please note that 100 g is not a very large portion and should not be exceeded.

- **Vegetables that grow below ground** – onions, beetroot, carrots, parsnip, turnip, celeriac
- **Some varieties of melon** – cantaloupe, watermelon
- **Some fruit** – apples, pears, peaches, plums, orange, pineapple, mango
- **Some berries** – blueberries, cherries
- **Some nuts and seeds** – hazelnuts, almonds, walnuts, pine nuts, sunflower seeds
- **Dairy** – whole milk, yoghurt
- **Beans and legumes** – peas and lupini beans

Foods that are high in carbohydrate

These foods should be eaten in very small quantities, or preferably avoided entirely by people suffering from insulin resistance. They contain high amounts of carbohydrate, usually 15 g per 100 g or over.

- **Nuts** – pistachios, cashews
- **Fruit** – grapes, bananas; all dried fruit, such as raisins and dates; all fruit juices and drinks
- **Vegetables that grow below ground** – potatoes and sweet potatoes
- **Beans and legumes** – kidney beans, lentils, black beans, chickpeas
- **Grains** – all grains, including breakfast cereals, bread, pasta, porridge.

The evidence

References

Introduction

1. Diabetes UK. Cost of diabetes. 15 Jan 2019. www.diabetes.co.uk/cost-of-diabetes.html and Diabetes prevalence. 15 jan 2019. www.diabetes.co.uk/diabetes-prevalence.html (accessed 28 June 2020)
2. NHS England. Musculoskeletal conditions. www.england.nhs.uk/ourwork/clinical-policy/ltc/our-work-on-long-term-conditions/musculoskeletal/ (accessed 28 June 2020) and Fibromyalgia. www.nhs.uk/conditions/fibromyalgia/ (accessed 4 July 2020)
3. Mental Health Foundation. Mental health statistics: UK and worldwide. www.mentalhealth.org.uk/statistics/mental-health-statistics-uk-and-worldwide (accessed 28 June 2020)
4. Arcidiacono B, Irritano S, Nocera A, et al. Insulin Resistance and Cancer Risk: An Overview of the Pathogenetic Mechanisms. *Experimental Diabetes Research* 2012; 2012: article ID 789174.
5. Boyd DB. Insulin and Cancer. *Integr Cancer Ther* 2003; 2(4): 315-329.
6. Crawford A. Increasing evidence of a strong connection between sugar and cancer. *Medical Xpress* Weill Cornell Medical College. March 20, 2019. https://medicalxpress.com/news/2019-03-evidence-strong-sugar-cancer.html (accessed 3.7.2020)
7. Centers for Disease Control and Prevention. Adult obesity prevalence maps. www.cdc.gov/obesity/data/prevalence-maps.html and Adult obesity facts www.cdc.gov/obesity/data/adult.html (accessed 28 June 2020)

8. Non-alcohol fatty liver disease (NAFLD), NHS England www.nhs.uk/conditions/non-alcoholic-fatty-liver-disease/ (accessed 28 June 2020)
9. Snel M, Jonker JT, Schoones J, Lamb H, et al. Ectopic fat and insulin resistance: pathophysiology and effect of diet and lifestyle interventions. *International Journal of Encocrinology* 2012; Article ID: 983814. insulin-resistance-and-ectopic-fat-a-diabetes-management.pdf
10. Cai J, Xu M, Zhang X, Li H. Innate Immune Signaling in Nonalcoholic Fatty Liver Disease and Cardio-vascular Diseases. *Annual Review of Pathology: Mechanisms of Disease*. 2018; 14: 153-184.

Chapter 1: What is insulin resistance?

1. Crescenzo R, Bianco F, Mazzoli A, Giacco A, Liverini G, Iossa S. Mitochondrial efficiency and insulin resistance. *Front Physiol* 2015; 5: 512. doi:10.3389/fphys.2014.00512
2. Sivitz WI, Yorek MA. Mitochondrial dysfunction in diabetes: from molecular mechanisms to functional significance and therapeutic opportunities. *Antioxidants & Redox Signaling* 2010; 12(4): 537–577.
3. De La Cruz C S, Kang M-J. Mitochondrial Dysfunction and Damage Associated Molecular Patterns (DAMPs) in Chronic Inflammatory Diseases. *Mitochondrion* 2018: 41: 37-44.
4. Forrester SJ, Kikuchi DS, Hernandes MS, et al. Reactive Oxygen Species in Metabolic and Inflammatory Signalling. *Circulation Research* 2018; 122: 877–902. doi.org/10.1161/CIRCRESAHA.117.311401
5. Lacourt TE, Vichaya EG, Chiu GS, Dantzer R, Heijnen CJ. The High Costs of Low-Grade Inflammation: Persistent Fatigue as a Consequence of Reduced Cellular-Energy Availability and Non-adaptive Energy Expenditure. *Frontiers in Behavioral Neuroscience* 2018; 12: 78. doi.org/10.3389/fnbeh.2018.00078

Chapter 2: What causes insulin resistance?

1. Finucane OM, Lynch CL, Murphy AM, Reynolds CM, et al. Monounsaturated fatty acid-enriched high-fat diets impede adipose NLRP3 inflammasome-mediated IL-1β secretion and

insulin resistance despite obesity. *Diabetes* 2015; 64(6): 2116-2128.
2. Patterson E, Wall R, Fitzgerald GF, et al. Health Implications of High Dietary Omega-6 Polyunsaturated Fatty Acids. *J Nutr Metab* 2012; 2012: 539426. doi: 10.1155/2012/539426
3. DiNicolantonio JJ, O'Keefe JH. Importance of maintaining a low omega–6/omega–3 ratio for reducing inflammation. *Open Heart* 2018; 5(2): e000946. doi: 10.1136/openhrt-2018-000946
4. Riccardi G, Giacco R, Rivellese AA. Dietary fat, insulin sensitivity and the metabolic syndrome. *Clin Nutr.* 2004;23(4):447–456. doi:10.1016/j.clnu.2004.02.006
5. Russo GL. Dietary n-6 and n-3 polyunsaturated fatty acids: from biochemistry to clinical implications in cardiovascular prevention. *Biochem Pharmacol* 2009; 77(6): 937-946. doi: 10.1016/j.bcp.2008.10.020.
6. Simopoulos A. An increase in the omega-6/omega-3 Fatty Acid Ratio Increases the Risk for Obesity. *Nutrients* 2016; 8(3): 128.
7. Simopoulos AP. The importance of the ratio of omega-6/omega-3 essential fatty acids. *Biomed Pharmacother* 2002; 56(8): 365-379.
8. Simopoulos AP. The importance of the omega-6/omega-3 fatty acid ratio in cardiovascular disease and other chronic diseases. *Exp Biol Med* 2008; 233(6): 674-688. doi: 10.3181/0711-MR-311.
9. Castañer O, Fitó M, López-Sabater M, Poulsen H, et al. The effect of olive oil polyphenols on anti-bodies against oxidized LDL. A randomized clinical trial. *Clinical Nutrition* 2011; 30: 490-493. doi: 10.1016/j.clnu.2011.01.013.
10. Cocchi M, Tonello L, Martínez J, Lercker G, Caramia G. Extra virgin olive oil and oleic acid. *Nutricion Clinica y Dietetica Hospitalaria* 2009; 29(3): 12-24.
11. George ES, Marshall S, Mayr HL, et al. The effect of high-polyphenol extra virgin olive oil on cardiovascular risk factors: A systematic review and meta-analysis. *Crit Rev Food Sci Nutr* 2019; 59(17): 2772–2795. doi:10.1080/10408398.2018.1470491
12. Hernáez Á, Fernández-Castillejo S, Farràs M, et al. Olive oil polyphenols enhance high-density lipo-protein function in humans: a randomized controlled trial. *Arterioscler Thromb Vasc Biol* 2014; 34(9): 2115–2119. doi:10.1161/ATVBAHA.114.303374
13. Schwingshackl L, Lampousi A, Portillo M, et al. Olive oil in the prevention and management of type 2 diabetes mellitus: a

systematic review and meta-analysis of cohort studies and intervention trials. *Nutr & Diabetes* 2017; 7: e262. doi.org/10.1038/nutd.2017.12

14. de Kort S, Keszthelyi D, Masclee AA. Leaky gut and diabetes mellitus: what is the link? *Obes Rev* 2011; 12(6): 449–458. doi:10.1111/j.1467-789X.2010.00845.x

15. Larsen N, Vogensen FK, van den Berg FWJ, et al. Gut microbiota in human adults with type 2 diabetes differs from non-diabetic adults. *PLoS ONE* 2010; 5(2): article e9085.

16. Thaiss CA, Levy M, Grosheva I, Zheng D, et al. Hyperglycemia drives intestinal barrier dysfunction and risk for enteric infection. *Science* 2018; 359(6382): 1376-1383. doi: 10.1126/science.aar3318

17. Zietek T, Rath E. Inflammation Meets Metabolic Disease: Gut Feeling Mediated by GLP-1. *Frontiers in Immunology* 2016; 7: 154. doi.org/10.3389/fimmu.2016.00154

18. Borghouts LB, Keizer HA. Exercise and insulin sensitivity: a review. *Int J Sports Med* 2000; 21(1): 1–12. doi:10.1055/s-2000-8847

19. Venkatasamy VV, Pericherla S, Manthuruthil S, Mishra S, Hanno R. Effect of Physical activity on Insulin Resistance, Inflammation and Oxidative Stress in Diabetes Mellitus. *Journal of Clinical and Diagnostic Research* 2013; 7(8): 1764–1766.

20. Dimitrov S, Hulteng E, Hong S. Inflammation and exercise: Inhibition of monocytic intracellular TNF production by acute exercise via β2-adrenergic activation. *Brain, Behavior and Immunity* 2017; 61: 60-68.

21. Costa RJS, Snipe RMJ, Kitic CM, Gibson PR. Systematic review: exercise-induced gastrointestinal syndrome-implications for health and intestinal disease. *Alimentary Pharmacology & Therapeutics* 2017; 46: 246-265. doi: 10.1111/apt.14157

22. Chiolero A, Faeh D, Paccaud F, Cornuz J. Consequences of smoking for body weight, body fat distribution, and insulin resistance. *American Journal of Clinical Nutrition* 2008; 87(4): 801–809. doi.org/10.1093/ajcn/87.4.801

23. Kapoor D, Jones TH. Smoking and hormones in health and endocrine disorders. *European Journal of Endocrinology* 2005; 152(4): 491-499. doi.org/10.1530/eje.1.01867

24. Rönnemaa T, Rönnemaa EM, Puukka P, et al. Smoking Is Independently Associated With High Plasma Insulin Levels in

Nondiabetic Men. *Diabetes Care* 1996; 19(11): 1229-1232. doi.org/10.2337/diacare.19.11.1229

25. Willi C, Bodenmann P, Ghali WA, et al. Active smoking and the risk of type 2 diabetes: a systematic review and meta-analysis. *JAMA* 2007; 298(22): 2654-2664.

26. Song MA, Reisinger SA, Freudenheim JL, et al. Effects of Electronic Cigarette Constituents on the Human Lung: A Pilot Clinical Trial. *Cancer Prev Res* 2020; 13(2): 145-152. doi:10.1158/1940-6207.CAPR-19-0400

27. Scott A, Lugg ST, Aldridge K, et al. Pro-inflammatory effects of e-cigarette vapour condensate on human alveolar macrophages. *Thorax* 2018; 73: 1161-1169.

28. Levy M, Kolodziejczyk AA, Thaiss CA, Elinav E. Dysbiosis and the immune system. *Nat Rev Immunol* 2017; 17(4): 219–232. doi:10.1038/nri.2017.7

Chapter 3: How do I know if I have insulin resistance?

1. Martin ET, Kaye KS, Knott C, Nguyen H. Diabetes and Risk of Surgical Site Infection: A Systematic Review and Meta-analysis. *Infect Control Hosp Epidemiol* 2016; 37(1): 88-99. doi: 10.1017/ice.2015.249.

2. Andersen CJ, Murphy KE, Fernandez ML. Impact of Obesity and Metabolic Syndrome on Immunity. *Adv Nutr* 2016; 7(1): 66–75. doi: 10.3945/an.115.010207

3. NHS England. Overview. High blood pressure (hypertension) www.nhs.uk/conditions/high-blood-pressure-hypertension/ (accessed 3 July 2020)

Chapter 4: What are the consequences of insulin resistance?

1. Fernandez-Morera L, Rodriguez-Rodero S, et al. The Possible Role of Epigenetics in Gestational Diabetes: Cause, Consequence, or Both. *Obstetrics and Gynecology International* 2010; 2010: Article ID 605163. doi.org/10.1155/2010/605163

2. Franzago M, Fraticelli F, Stuppia L, Vitacolonna E. Nutrigenetics,

epigenetics and gestational diabetes: consequences in mother and child. *Epigenetics* 2019; 14(3): 215–235. doi:10.1080/15592294.2019.1582277

3. Rhee EJ, Lee WY, Cho YK, Kim BI, Sung KC. Hyperinsulinemia and the development of nonalcoholic fatty liver disease in nondiabetic adults. *Am J Med* 2011; 124(1): 69–76. doi:10.1016/j.amjmed.2010.08.012

4. Santoleri D, Titchenell PM. Resolving the Paradox of Hepatic Insulin Resistance. *CMGH Journal* 2018; 7(2): 447-456. doi:10.1016/j.jcmgh.2018.10.016

5. Brenta G. Why can insulin resistance be a natural consequence of thyroid dysfunction. *Journal of Thyroid Research* 2011; 2011: Article ID 152850. doi.org/10.4061/2011/152850

6. Crunkhorn S, Patti ME. Links between thyroid hormone action, oxidative metabolism, and diabetes risk? *Thyroid* 2008; 18(2): 227-237. doi:10.1089/thy.2007.0249

7. Gierach M, et al. Insulin resistance and thyroid disorders. *Endokrynol Pol* 2014; 65(1): 70-76. doi: 10.5603/EP.2014.0010.

8. Jurjus A, Eid A, Al Kattar S, et al. Inflammatory bowel disease, colorectal cancer and type 2 diabetes mellitus: The links. *BBA Clin* 2016; 5: 16–24. doi: 10.1016/j.bbacli.2015.11.002

9. Piper MS, Saad RJ. Diabetes Mellitus and the Colon. *Current Treatment Options in Gastroenterology* 2017; 15(4): 460–474. doi.org/10.1007/s11938-017-0151-1

10. Pappolla MA, Manchikanti L, Andersen CR, et al. Is insulin resistance the cause of fibromyalgia? A preliminary report. *PLOS ONE* 2019; 14 (5): e0216079. doi: 10.1371/journal.pone.0216079

11. Sinaii N, Cleary SD, Ballweg ML, Nieman LK, Stratton P. High rates of autoimmune and endocrine disorders, fibromyalgia, chronic fatigue syndrome and atopic diseases among women with endometriosis: a survey analysis. *Hum Reprod* 2002; 17(10): 2715-2724.

12. Minerbi A, Gonzalez E, Brereton NJB, et al. Altered microbiome composition in individuals with fibromyalgia. *Pain* 2019; 160(11): 2589-2602. doi: 10.1097/j.pain.0000000000001640.

13. Han L, Ji L, Chang J, et al. Peripheral neuropathy is associated with insulin resistance independent of metabolic syndrome. *Diabetol Metab Syndr* 2015; 7: 14. doi: 10.1186/s13098-015-0010-y

14. Stino AM, Smith AG. Peripheral neuropathy in prediabetes and the metabolic syndrome. *J Diabetes Investig*. 2017; 8(5): 646–655. doi: 10.1111/jdi.12650
15. Wu Y, He H, Yu K, et al. The association between serum uric acid levels and insulin resistance and secretion in prediabetes mellitus: A cross-sectional study. *Ann Clin Lab Sci* 2019; 49(2): 218-223.
16. Malhotra A. Saturated fat is not the major issue. *Br Med J* 2013; 347: f6340.
17. Bowers LW, Rossi EL, O'Flanagan [initials?], et al. The role of the insulin/IGF system in cancer: lessons learned from clinical trials and the energy balance-cancer link. *Front Endocrinol* 2015; 6: 77. doi:10.3389/fendo.2015.00077
18. Cohen DH and LeRoith D. Obesity, type 2 diabetes, and cancer: the insulin and IGF connection. Endocrine-Related Cancer. 2012; 19(5): F27-F45.
19. Grimberg A. Mechanisms by which IGF-I may promote cancer. *Cancer Biology & Therapy* 2003; 2(6): 630–635.
20. Port AM, Ruth MR, Istfan NW. Fructose consumption and cancer: is there a connection? *Curr Opin Endocrinol Diabetes Obes* 2012;19(5): 367-374. doi: 10.1097/MED.0b013e328357f0cb.
21. Seyfried TN. Cancer as a mitochondrial metabolic disease. Hypothesis and Theory Article. *Frontiers in Cell and Developmental Biology* 2015; 3: 43. doi.org/10.3389/fcell.2015.00043
22. Seyfried TN, Flores RE, et al. Cancer as a metabolic disease: implications for novel therapeutics. *Carcinogenesis* 2014; 35(3): 515-527.
23. Seyfried TN, Shelton L M. Cancer as a metabolic disease. *Nutr Metab* 2010; 7: 7. doi.org/10.1186/1743-7075-7-7
24. Tan-Shalaby J. Ketogenic Diets and Cancer: Emerging Evidence. *Fed Pract* 2017: 34(Suppl 1): 37S-42S.
25. Alzheimer's Research UK. Dementia Statistics Hub. Prevalence. www.dementiastatistics.org/statistics-about-dementia/prevalence/ (accessed 3 July 2020); Alz-heimer's Research UK. Dementia Statistics Hub. Global Prevalence. 5 July 2018. www.dementiastatistics.org/statistics/global-prevalence/ (accessed 3 July 20); Alzheimer's Research UK. Make breakthroughs possible. Risk factors. www.alzheimersresearchuk.org/about-

dementia/types-of-dementia/alzheimers-disease/risk-factors/ (accessed 3 July 2020); NHS England. Alzheimers disease. Overview. www.nhs.uk/conditions/alzheimers-disease/ (accessed 3 July 2020); World Health Organization. Dementia. Key facts. 19 Sep 2019. www.who.int/news-room/fact-sheets/detail/dementia (accessed 3 July 2020)
26. Arnold SE, Arvanitakis Z, Macauley-Rambach SL, Koenig AM, et al. Brain insulin resistance in type 2 diabetes and Alzheimer disease: concepts and conundrums. *Nat Rev Neurol* 2018; 14: 168–181. doi.org/10.1038/nrneurol.2017.185
27. Berger AL. Insulin resistance and reduced brain glucose metabolism in the aetiology of Alzheimer's disease. *Journal of Insulin Resistance* 2016; 1(1): 7.
28. Blázquez E, Velázquez E, Hurtado-Carneiro V, Ruiz-Albusac JM. Insulin in the brain: Its pathophysiological implications for states related with central insulin resistance, type 2 diabetes and Alzheimer's disease. *Front Endocrinol* 2014; 5: 161.
29. Cunnane SC, Courchesne-Loyer A, St-Pierre V, Vandenberghe C, et al. Can ketones compensate for deteriorating brain glucose uptake during aging? Implications for the risk and treatment of Alzheimer's disease. *Ann NY Acad Sci* 2016;1367(1): 12-20. doi: 10.1111/nyas.12999.
30. Ede G. Diagnosis:Diet. Avoiding Alzheimer's Disease Could Be Easier Than You Think. Science shines bright light on root cause of memory problems. *PsychologyToday* Posted 7 Sep 2016. (www.psychologytoday.com/us/blog/diagnosis-diet/201609/avoiding-alzheimer-s-disease-could-be-easier-you-think – accessed 24 June 2020)
31. Ferreira LSS, Fernandes CS, Vieira MNN, De Felice FG. Insulin Resistance in Alzheimer's Disease. *Front Neurosci* 2018; 12: 830. doi: 10.3389/fnins.2018.00830
32. Luchsinger JA. Adiposity, hyperinsulinemia, diabetes and Alzheimer's disease. An epidemiological perspective. *European Journal of Pharmacology* 2008; 585(1): 119-129.
33. Plum L, Schubert M, Brüning JC. The role of insulin receptor signaling in the brain. *Trends Endocrinol Metab* 2005; 16(2): 59–65.
34. Mental Health Foundation. Mental health statistics: depression. www.mentalhealth.org.uk/statistics/mental-health-statistics-

depression (accessed 28 June 2020)
35. Faig MA, Dada T. Diabetes Type 4: A Paradigm Shift in the Understanding of Glaucoma, the Brain Specific Diabetes and the candidature of insulin as a therapeutic agent. *Curr Mol Med* 2017; 17(1): 46-59. doi: 10.2174/1566524017666170206153415.
36. Dada T. Is Glaucoma a Neurodegeneration caused by Central Insulin Resistance: Diabetes Type 4?. *Journal of Current Glaucoma Practice* 2017; 11(3): 77-79. doi: 10.5005/jp-journals-10028-1228
37. Chen X, Rong SS, Xu Q, Tang FY, et al. Diabetes mellitus and risk of age-related macular degeneration: a systematic review and meta-analysis. *PloS One* 2014; 9(9): e108196. doi.org/10.1371/journal.pone.0108196
38. Chopra R, Chander A, Jacob JJ. Ocular associations of metabolic syndrome. *Indian J Endocrinol Metab* 2012; 16(Suppl1): S6–S11. doi: 10.4103/2230-8210.94244
39. Karaca C, Karaca Z. Beyond Hyperglycemia, Evidence for Retinal Neurodegeneration in Metabolic Syndrome. *Invest Ophthalmol Vis Sci* 2018; 59(3): 1360-1367. doi:10.1167/iovs.17-23376
40. Lee CS, Larson EB, Gibbons LE, et al. Associations between recent and established ophthalmic conditions and risk of Alzheimer's disease. *Alzheimer's & Dementia* 2019; 15(1): 34-41. doi.org/10.1016/j.jalz.2018.06.2856
41. Mbata O, El-Magd NFA, El-Remessy AB. Obesity, metabolic syndrome and diabetic retinopathy: Beyond hyperglycemia. *World J Diabetes* 2017; 8(7): 317–329. doi: 10.4239/wjd.v8.i7.317
42. Ming-Shan He, Fang-Ling Chang, Hong-Zin Lin, Jung-Lun Wu, Tsung-Cheng Hsieh, Yuan-Chieh Lee. The Association Between Diabetes and Age-Related Macular Degeneration Among the Elderly in Taiwan. *Diabetes Care* 2018; 41(10): 2202-2211. doi: 10.2337/dc18-0707

Chapter 5: How can I reverse insulin resistance?

1. Bhanpuri NH, Hallberg SJ, Williams PT, et al. Cardiovascular disease risk factor responses to a type 2 diabetes care model including nutritional ketosis induced by sustained carbohydrate restriction at 1 year: an open label, non-randomized, controlled

study. *Cardiovasc Diabetol* 2018; 17(1): 56.
doi: 10.1186/s12933-018-0698-8
2. Masino SA, Ruskin DN. Ketogenic diets and pain. *Journal of Child Neurology* 2013; 28(8): 993–1001.
3. Newman JC, Verdin E. β-hydroxybutyrate: much more than a metabolite. *Diabetes Res Clin Pract* 2014; 106(2): 173–181. doi:10.1016/j.diabres.2014.08.009
4. Pinto A, Bonucci A, Maggi E, Corsi M, Businaro, R. (2018). Anti-Oxidant and Anti-Inflammatory Activity of Ketogenic Diet: New Perspectives for Neuroprotection in Alzheimer's Disease. *Antioxidants* 2018; 7(5): 63.
5. Shimazu T, Hirschey MD, Newman J, He W, et al. 2013). Suppression of oxidative stress by β-hydroxybutyrate, an endogenous histone deacetylase inhibitor. *Science* 2013; 339(6116): 211–214.
6. Youm YH, Nguyen KY, Grant R W et al (2015). The ketone metabolite β-hydroxybutyrate blocks NLRP3 inflammasome-mediated inflammatory disease. *Nat Med* 2015; 21(3):263-269. doi: 10.1038/nm.3804.
7. Goldberg EL, Molony RD, Kudo E, et al. Ketogenic diet activates protective γδ T cell responses against influenza virus infection. *Science Immunology* 2019; 4(41): eaav2026.
doi: 10.1126/sciimmunol.aav2026
8. Ho KL, Zhang L, Wagg C, Al Batran R, et al. Increased ketone body oxidation provides additional energy for the failing heart without improving cardiac efficiency. *Cardiovascular Research* 2019; 115(11): 1606–1616. doi.org/10.1093/cvr/cvz045
9. Miller VJ, Villamena FA, Volek JS. Nutritional Ketosis and Mitohormesis: Potential Implications for Mitochondrial Function and Human Health. *Journal of Nutrition and Metabolism* 2018; 2018:Article ID 5157645. doi.org/10.1155/2018/5157645
10. Parker BA, Walton CM, Carr ST, et al. β-Hydroxybutyrate Elicits Favorable Mitochondrial Changes in Skeletal Muscle. *Int J Mol Sci* 2018; 19(8): 2247. doi:10.3390/ijms19082247
11. Do MH, Lee E, Oh MJ, Kim Y, Park HY. High-glucose or -fructose diets cause changes of the gut microbiota and metabolic disorders in mice without body weight change. *Nutrients* 2018; 10(6): 761.
12. Yang Q. Gain weight by "going diet?" Artificial sweeteners and the

The evidence

neurobiology of sugar cravings: Neuroscience 2010. *Yale Journal of Biology and Medicine* 2010; 83(2): 101–108.
13. Suez J, Korem T, Zeevi D, et al. Artificial sweeteners induce glucose intolerance by altering the gut microbiota. *Nature* 2014; 514(7521): 181–186. doi:10.1038/nature13793
14. Public Health Collaboration. Sugar Equivalent Infographics courtesy of Dr David Unwin. https://phcuk.org/sugar/ (accessed 28 June 2020)
15. Aksungar FB, Topkaya AE, Akyildiz M et al. Interleukin-6, C-reactive protein and biochemical parameters during prolonged intermittent fasting. *Ann Nutr Metab* 2007; 51(1): 88-95.
16. Alirezaei M, Kemball CC, Flynn C T, et al. Short-term fasting induces profound neuronal autophagy. *Autophagy* 2010; 6(6): 702–710. doi: 10.4161/auto.6.6.12376
17. Anton SD, Moehl K, Donahoo WT, et al. Flipping the Metabolic Switch: Understanding and Applying Health Benefits of Fasting. *Obesity* 2018; 26(2): 254–268. doi: 10.1002/oby.22065
18. Blackman MR, Sorkin JD, Münzer T, et al. Growth hormone and sex steroid administration in healthy aged women and men: a randomized controlled trial. *JAMA* 2002; 288(18): 2282-2292.
19. Furmli S, Elmasry R, Ramos M, Fung J. Therapeutic use of intermittent fasting for people with type 2 diabetes as an alternative to insulin. *Br Med J* 2018; 2018: pii: bcr-2017-221854. doi: 10.1136/bcr-2017-221854.
20. Ganesan K, Habboush Y, Sultan S. Intermittent Fasting: The Choice for a Healthier Lifestyle. *Cureus* 2018; 10(7): e2947. doi: 10.7759/cureus.2947
21. Halberg N, Henriksen M, Söderhamn N, et al. Effect of intermittent fasting and refeeding on insulin action in healthy men. *J Appl Physiol* 2005; 99(6): 2128-2136.
22. Hartman ML, Veldhuis JD, Johnson ML, et al. Augmented growth hormone (GH) secretory burst frequency and amplitude mediate enhanced GH secretion during a two-day fast in normal men. *J Clin Endocrinol Metab* 1992; 74(4): 757-765.
23. Harvie MN, Pegington M, Mattson MP. The effects of intermittent or continuous energy restriction on weight loss and metabolic disease risk markers: a randomised trial in young overweight women. *Int J Obes* 2011; 35(5): 714–727. doi: 10.1038/ijo.2010.171

24. Heilbronn LK, Smith SR, Martin CK, et al. Alternate-day fasting in nonobese subjects: effects on body weight, body composition, and energy metabolism. *Am J Clin Nutr* 2005; 81(1): 69-73.
25. Ho KY, Veldhuis JD, Johnson ML, et al. Fasting enhances growth hormone secretion and amplifies the complex rhythms of growth hormone secretion in man. *J Clin Invest* 1988; 81(4): 968–975. doi: 10.1172/JCI113450
26. Johnson JB, Summer W, Cutler RG, et al. Alternate day calorie restriction improves clinical findings and reduces markers of oxidative stress and inflammation in overweight adults with moderate asthma. *Free Radic Biol Med* 2007; 42(5): 665-474.
27. Johnstone A. Fasting for weight loss: an effective strategy or latest dieting trend? *Int J Obes* 2015; 39(5): 727-733. doi: 10.1038/ijo.2014.214.
28. Kahleova H, Belinova L, Malinska H, et al. Eating two larger meals a day (breakfast and lunch) is more effective than six smaller meals in a reduced-energy regimen for patients with type 2 diabetes: a randomised crossover study. *Diabetologia* 2014; 57(8): 1552-1560. doi: 10.1007/s00125-014-3253-5.
29. Martin B, Mattson MP, Maudsley S. Caloric restriction and intermittent fasting: Two potential diets for successful brain aging. *Ageing Res Rev* 2006; 5(3): 332–353. doi: 10.1016/j.arr.2006.04.002
30. Mattson MP, Moehl K, et al. Intermittent metabolic switching, neuroplasticity and brain health. *Nat Rev Neurosci* 2018; 19(2): 63–80. doi: 10.1038/nrn.2017.156
31. Mattson MP, Longo VD, Harvie M. Impact of Intermittent Fasting on Health and Disease Processes. *Aging Res Rev* 2017; 39: 46-58.
32. Moro T, Tinsley G, Bianco A. Effects of eight weeks of time-restricted feeding (16/8) on basal metabolism, maximal strength, body composition, inflammation, and cardiovascular risk factors in resistance-trained males. *J Transl Med* 2016; 14: 290. doi: 10.1186/s12967-016-1044-0
33. Persynaki A, Karras S, Pichard C. Unraveling the metabolic health benefits of fasting related to religious beliefs: A narrative review. *Nutrition* 2017; 35: 14-20. doi: 10.1016/j.nut.2016.10.005.
34. Rothschild J, Hoddy K, Jambazian P, Varady KA. Time-restricted feeding and risk of metabolic disease: a review of human and

animal studies. *Nutrition Reviews* 2014; 72(5): 308–318.
35. Rudman D, Feller AG, Nagraj HS, et al. Effects of human growth hormone in men over 60 years old. *N Engl J Med* 1990; 323(1): 1-6.
36. Shariatpanahi ZV, Shariatpanahi MV, et al. Effect of Ramadan fasting on some indices of insulin resistance and components of the metabolic syndrome in healthy male adults. *Br J Nutr* 2008; 100(1): 147-151.
37. Sievert K, Hussain SM, Page MJ, et al. Effect of breakfast on weight and energy intake: systematic review and meta-analysis of randomised controlled trials. *Br Med J* 2019; 364: l42.
38. Zhu Y, Yan Y, Gius DR, Vassilopoulos A. Metabolic regulation of Sirtuins upon fasting and the implication for cancer. *Curr Opin Oncol* 2013; 25(6): 630-636.
doi: 10.1097/01.cco.0000432527.49984.a3.
39. Diabetes.co.uk. Vitamin C linked to reduced glucose levels in type 2 diabetes. 11 Feb 2019. www.diabetes.co.uk/news/2019/feb/vitamin-c-linked-to-reduced-glucose-levels-in-type-2-diabetes-95348957.html (accessed 28 June 2020)
40. Diabetes.co.uk. Vitamin D and diabetes. 15 Jan 2019. www.diabetes.co.uk/food/vitamin-d.html (accessed 28 June 2020)
41. Dakhale GN, Chaudhari HV, Shrivastava M. Supplementation of Vitamin C Reduces Blood Glucose and Improves Glycosylated Hemoglobin in Type 2 Diabetes Mellitus: A Randomized, Double-Blind Study. *Advances in Pharmacological and Pharmaceutical Sciences* 2011; 2011: Article ID 195271
doi.org/10.1155/2011/195271
42. Huerta MG, Roemmich JM, et al. Magnesium Deficiency Is Associated With Insulin Resistance in Obese Children. *Diabetes Care* 2005; 28(5): 1175-1181.
43. Kayaniyil S, Vieth R, Retnakaran R, et al. Association of vitamin D with insulin resistance and beta-cell dysfunction in subjects at risk for type 2 diabetes. *Diabetes Care* 2010; 33(6): 1379-1381.
doi: 10.2337/dc09-2321.
44. Kostov K. Effects of Magnesium Deficiency on Mechanisms of Insulin Resistance in Type 2 Diabetes: Focusing on the Processes of Insulin Secretion and Signaling. *Int J Mol Sci* 2019; 20(6): 1351.
doi: 10.3390/ijms20061351
45. Lv WS, Zhao WJ, Gong SL, et al. Serum 25-hydroxyvitamin D levels

and peripheral neuropathy in patients with type 2 diabetes: a systematic review and meta-analysis. *J Endocrinol Invest* 2015; 38: 513–518. doi.org/10.1007/s40618-014-0210-6

46. Montero D, Walther G, Stehouwer CDA, et al. Effect of antioxidant vitamin supplementation on endothelial function in type 2 diabetes mellitus: a systematic review and meta-analysis of randomized controlled trials. *Obesity Reviews* 2014; 15(2): 107–116. doi: 10.1111/obr.12114

47. Wilson R, Willis J, Gearry R, et al. Inadequate Vitamin C Status in Prediabetes and Type 2 Diabetes Mellitus: Associations with Glycaemic Control, Obesity, and Smoking. *Nutrients* 2017; 9(9): 997. doi: 10.3390/nu9090997

48. Szymczak-Pajor I, Śliwińska A. Analysis of Association between Vitamin D Deficiency and Insulin Resistance. *Nutrients* 2019; 11(4): 794. doi.org/10.3390/nu11040794

49. Calvano A, Izuora K, Oh EC, Ebersole JL, Lyons TJ, Basu A. Dietary berries, insulin resistance and type 2 diabetes: an overview of human feeding trials. *Food & Function* 2019; 10(10): 6227–6243. doi.org/10.1039/c9fo01426h

50. Joseph SV, Edirisinghe I, Burton-Freeman BM. Berries: anti-inflammatory effects in humans. *J Agric Food Chem* 2014; 62(18): 3886-3903. doi: 10.1021/jf4044056.

51. Martineau LC, Couture A, Spoor D, et al. Anti-diabetic properties of the Canadian lowbush blueberry Vaccinium angustifolium Ait. *Phytomedicine* 2006; 13(9–10): 612-623.

52. Stull AJ. (2016). Blueberries' Impact on Insulin Resistance and Glucose Intolerance. *Antioxidants* 2016; 5(4): 44. doi.org/10.3390/antiox5040044

53. Fromentin C, Tomé D, Nau F, et al. Dietary proteins contribute little to glucose production, even under optimal gluconeogenic conditions in healthy humans. *Diabetes* 2013; 62(5): 1435–1442. doi:10.2337/db12-1208

54. Gannon MC, Nuttall JA, Damberg G, Gupta V, Nuttall FQ. Effect of protein ingestion on the glucose appearance rate in people with type 2 diabetes. *J Clin Endocrinol Metab* 2001; 86(3): 1040–1047. doi:10.1210/jcem.86.3.7263

55. Prokopieva VD, Yarygina EG, Bokhan NA, Ivanova SA. Use of Carnosine for Oxidative Stress Reduction in Different

Pathologies. *Oxidative Medicine and Cellular Longevity* 2016: 2939087. doi.org/10.1155/2016/2939087

56. Marí M, Morales A, Colell A, García-Ruiz C, Fernández-Checa JC. Mitochondrial glutathione, a key survival antioxidant. *Antioxidants & Redox Signaling* 2009; 11(11): 2685–2700. doi.org/10.1089/ARS.2009.2695
57. Saini R. Coenzyme Q10: The essential nutrient. *Journal of Pharmacy & Bioallied Sciences* 2011; 3(3): 466–467. doi.org/10.4103/0975-7406.84471
58. Cararo JH, Streck EL, Schuck PF, Ferreira G. Carnosine and Related Peptides: Therapeutic Potential in Age-Related Disorders. *Aging and Disease* 2015; 6(5): 369–379. doi.org/10.14336/AD.2015.0616
59. Quinzii CM, Hirano M. Coenzyme Q and mitochondrial disease. *Developmental Disabilities Research Reviews* 2010; 16(2): 183–188. doi.org/10.1002/ddrr.108
60. Adeva-Andany M, Souto-Adeva G, Ameneiros-Rodríguez E, Fernández-Fernández C, Donapetry-García C, Domínguez-Montero A. Insulin resistance and glycine metabolism in humans. *Amino Acids* 2018; 50(1): 11–27. doi:10.1007/s00726-017-2508-0
61. Reid G, Jass J, Sebulsky MT, McCormick JK. Potential uses of probiotics in clinical practice. *Clin Microbiol Rev* 2003; 16(4): 658–672. doi:10.1128/cmr.16.4.658-672.2003
62. Spaiser SJ, Culpepper T, Nieves C Jr, et al. Lactobacillus gasseri KS-13, Bifidobacterium bifidum G9-1, and Bifidobacterium longum MM-2 Ingestion Induces a Less Inflammatory Cytokine Profile and a Po-tentially Beneficial Shift in Gut Microbiota in Older Adults: A Randomized, Double-Blind, Placebo-Controlled, Crossover Study. *J Am Coll Nutr* 2015; 34(6): 459–469. doi:10.1080/07315724.2014.983249
63. BioCare. Probiotic research. www.biocare.co.uk/probiotic-research (accessed 28 June 2020)
64. Daniel K. Why broth is beautiful: essential roles for proline, glycine and gelatin. 18 June 2003. www.westonaprice.org/health-topics/why-broth-is-beautiful-essential-roles-for-proline-glycine-and-gelatin/ (accessed 28 June 2020)
65. Allen JM, Mailing LJ, Niemiro GM, et al. Exercise Alters Gut Microbiota Composition and Function in Lean and Obese Humans. *Med Sci Sports Exerc* 2018; 50(4): 747-757.

doi: 10.1249/MSS.0000000000001495.
66. Mailing LJ, Allen JM, Buford TW, et al. Exercise and the Gut Microbiome: A Review of the Evidence, Potential Mechanisms, and Implications for Human Health. *Exerc Sport Sci Rev* 2019; 47(2): 75-85. doi: 10.1249/JES.0000000000000183.
67. Monda V, Villano I, Messina A, et al. Exercise Modifies the Gut Microbiota with Positive Health Effects. *Oxid Med Cell Longev* 2017; 2017: 3831972. doi: 10.1155/2017/3831972
68. Costantini L, Molinari R, Farinon B, Merendino N. (2017). Impact of Omega-3 Fatty Acids on the Gut Microbiota. *International Journal of Molecular Sciences* 2017; 18(12): 2645.
69. Søgaard D, Lund MT, Scheuer CM, et al. High-intensity interval training improves insulin sensitivity in older individuals. *Acta Physiol.* 2018; 222(4): e13009. doi: 10.1111/apha.13009.
70. Diabetes.co.uk. HIIT fights insulin resistance in women at risk of type 2 diabetes. 17 August 2017. www.diabetes.co.uk/news/2017/aug/hiit-fights-insulin-resistance-in-women-at-risk-of-type-2-diabetes-98446049.html (accessed 28 June 2020)
71. Naik D, Thomas N. Yoga- a potential solution for diabetes and metabolic syndrome. *Indian Journal of Medical Research* 2015; 141(6): 753–756. doi: 10.4103/0971-5916.160689
72. Raveendran AV, Deshpandae A, Joshi SR. Therapeutic Role of Yoga in Type 2 Diabetes. *Endocrinology and Metabolism* 2018; 33(3): 307–317. doi: 10.3803/EnM.2018.33.3.307
73. Joslin Diabetes Center. Insulin resistance in the brain, behavioral disorders: Direct link found. *ScienceDaily* 2 March 2015. www.sciencedaily.com/releases/2015/03/150302121504.htm (accessed 14 February 2020)
74. Manpreet K, Sing S, Leslie M, et al. Brain and behavioral correlates of insulin resistance in youth with depression and obesity. *Hormones and Behavior* 2019; 108: 73-83.
75. Scott EM, Carpenter JS, Iorfino F, et al. What is the prevalence, and what are the clinical correlates, of insulin resistance in young people presenting for mental health care? A cross-sectional study. *Br Med J Open* 2019; 9: e025674.
doi: 10.1136/bmjopen-2018-025674
76. Silva NM, Lam MP, Soares CN, et al. Insulin resistance as a shared pathogenic mechanism between depression and type 2 diabetes.

The evidence

Front Psychiatry 2019; 10: 57. doi: 10.3389/fpsyt.2019.00057

77. Özalp Kizilay D, Yalin Sapmaz S, Sen S, et al. Insulin Resistance as Related to Psychiatric Disorders in Obese Children. *J Clin Res Pediatr Endocrinol* 2018; 10(4): 364–372. doi: 10.4274/jcrpe.0055

78. Wolf T, Tsenkova V, Ryff CD, Davidson RJ, Willette AA. Neural, Hormonal, and Cognitive Correlates of Metabolic Dysfunction and Emotional Reactivity. *Psychosomatic Medicine* 2018; 80(5): 452–459. doi.org/10.1097/PSY.0000000000000582

79. Rubin R. Exploring the Relationship Between Depression and Dementia. *JAMA* 2018; 320(10): 961–962. doi:10.1001/jama.2018.11154

80. Soontornniyomkij V, Lee EE, Jin H, Martin AS, et al. Clinical Correlates of Insulin Resistance in Chronic Schizophrenia: Relationship to Negative Symptoms. *Frontiers in Psychiatry* 2019; 10: 251. doi.org/10.3389/fpsyt.2019.00251

81. Jääskeläinen T, Knekt P, Suvisaari J, et al. Higher serum 25-hydroxyvitamin D concentrations are related to a reduced risk of depression. *British Journal of Nutrition* 2015; 113(9): 1418-1426. doi: 10.1017/S0007114515000689

82. Kerr DCR, Zava DT, Piper WT, Saturn SR, Frei B, Gombart AF. Associations between vitamin D levels and depressive Symptoms in healthy young adult women. *Psychiatry Research* 2015; 227(1): 46-51. doi: 10.1016/j.psychres.2015.02.016

83. Kiecolt-Glaser JK, Belury MA, Andridge R, Malarkey WB, Glaser R. Omega-3 supplementation lowers inflammation and anxiety in medical students: a randomized controlled trial. *Brain Behav Immun* 2011; 25(8): 1725–1734. doi:10.1016/j.bbi.2011.07.229

84. Su KP, Yang HT, Chang JP, et al. Eicosapentaenoic and docosahexaenoic acids have different effects on peripheral phospholipase A2 gene expressions in acute depressed patients. *Progress in Neuropsychopharmacology and Biological Psychiatry* 2018; 80(Pt C): 227-233. doi: 10.1016/j.pnpbp.2017.06.020. 2

85. Ginty AT, Conklin SM. Short-term supplementation of acute long-chain omega-3 polyunsaturated fatty acids may alter depression status and decrease symptomology among young adults with depression: A preliminary randomized and placebo controlled trial. *Psychiatry Research* 2015; 229(1-2): 485-489. doi: 10.1016/j.psychres.2015.05.072

86. Martins JG. EPA but not DHA appears to be responsible for the efficacy of omega-3 long chain polyunsaturated fatty acid supplementation in depression: evidence from a meta-analysis of randomized controlled trials. *Journal of the American College of Nutrition* 2009; 28(5): 525-542.
87. Martins JG, Bentsen H, Puri BK. Eicosapentaenoic acid appears to be the key omega-3 fatty acid component associated with efficacy in major depressive disorder: a critique of Bloch and Hannestad and updated meta-analysis. *Molecular Psychiatry* 2012; 17(12): 1144-1149; discussion 1163-1167.
88. Pratte MA, Nanavati KB, Young V, Morley CP. An alternative treatment for anxiety: a systematic review of human trial results reported for the Ayurvedic herb ashwagandha (Withania somnifera). *J Altern Complement Med* 2014; 20(12): 901–908. doi:10.1089/acm.2014.0177
89. Mirza B, Ikram H, Bilgrami S, Haleem DJ, Haleem MA. Neurochemical and behavioral effects of green tea (Camellia sinensis): a model study. *Pak J Pharm Sci* 2013; 26(3): 511–516.
90. Ideno Y, Hayashi K, Abe Y, et al. Blood pressure-lowering effect of Shinrin-yoku (Forest bathing): a systematic review and meta-analysis. *BMC Complementary Medicine and Therapies* 2017; 17: 409. doi: 10.1186/s12906-017-1912-z
91. Ohtsuka Y, Yabunaka N, Takayama S. Shinrin-yoku (forest-air bathing and walking) effectively decreases blood glucose levels in diabetic patients. *Int J Biometeorol* 1998; 41(3): 125-127.
92. Kuo M. How might contact with nature promote human health? Promising mechanisms and a possible central pathway. *Frontiers in Psychology* 25 August 2015. doi: 10.3389/fpsyg.2015.01093
93. Goyal M, Singh S, Sibinga EM, et al. Meditation programs for psychological stress and well-being: a systematic review and meta-analysis. *JAMA Intern Med* 2014; 174(3): 357-68. doi: 10.1001/jamainternmed.2013.13018.
94. Ong JC, Manber R, Segal Z, et al. A randomized controlled trial of mindfulness meditation for chronic insomnia. *Sleep* 2014; 37(9): 1553-1563. doi: 10.5665/sleep.4010.
95. Sinha SS, Jain AK, Tyagi S, et al. Effect of 6 Months of Meditation on Blood Sugar, Glycosylated Hemoglobin, and Insulin Levels in Patients of Coronary Artery Disease. *International Journal of Yoga*

2018; 11(2): 122–128. doi: 10.4103/ijoy.IJOY_30_17
96. Chen MC, Fang SH, Fang L. The effects of aromatherapy in relieving symptoms related to job stress among nurses. *Int J Nurs Pract* 2015; 21(1): 87–93. doi:10.1111/ijn.12229
97. Hwang E, Shin S. The effects of aromatherapy on sleep improvement: a systematic literature review and meta-analysis. *J Altern Complement Med* 2015; 21(2): 61–68. doi:10.1089/acm.2014.0113
98. Donga E, van Dijk M, van Dijk JG, et al. A single night of partial sleep deprivation induces insulin resistance in multiple metabolic pathways in healthy subjects. *J Clin Endocrinol Metab* 2010; 95(6): 2963–2968. doi:10.1210/jc.2009-2430
99. Ong DK, Mitchell SB, Barrett JS, et al. Manipulation of dietary short chain carbohydrates alters the pattern of gas production and genesis of symptoms in irritable bowel syndrome. *J Gastroenterol Hepatol* 2010; 25(8): 1366–1373. doi:10.1111/j.1440-1746.2010.06370.x
100. Barrett JS, Gibson PR. Fermentable oligosaccharides, disaccharides, monosaccharides and polyols (FODMAPs) and nonallergic food intolerance: FODMAPs or food chemicals? *Therapeutic Advanc-es in Gastroenterology* 2012; 5(4): 261–268. doi.org/10.1177/1756283X11436241
101. Casal S, Malheiro R, Sendas A, et al. Olive oil stability under deep-frying conditions. *Food and Chemical Toxicology* 2010; 48(10): 2972-2979. doi.org/10.1016/j.fct.2010.07.036

Chapter 6: Special considerations

1. NHS England. Salt: The facts. Eat well. www.nhs.uk/live-well/eat-well/salt-nutrition/ (accessed 4 July 2020)
2. Mente A, O'Donnell M, Rangarajan S, et al. Associations of urinary sodium excretion with cardiovascular events in individuals with and without hypertension: a pooled analysis of data from four studies. *Lancet* 2016; 388(10043): 465-475. doi:10.1016/S0140-6736(16)30467-6
3. Cardio Brief. International Experts Call Salt Guidelines Far Too Restrictive. 14 February 2017. www.cardiobrief.org/2017/02/14/

international-experts-call-salt-guidelines-far-too-restrictive/ (accessed 3 July 2020)
4. Kampmann U, Knorr S, Fuglsang J, Ovesen P. Determinants of Maternal Insulin Resistance during Pregnancy: An Updated Overview. *J Diabetes Res.* 2019; 2019: 5320156. doi:10.1155/2019/5320156
5. Ruiz-Palacios M, Ruiz-Alcaraz AJ, Sanchez-Campillo M, Larqué E. Role of Insulin in Placental Transport of Nutrients in Gestational Diabetes Mellitus. *Ann Nutr Metab.* 2017; 70(1): 16-25. doi:10.1159/000455904
6. Vega M, Mauro M, Williams Z. Direct toxicity of insulin on the human placenta and protection by metformin. *Fertil Steril.* 2019; 111(3): 489-496. e5. doi:10.1016/j.fertnstert.2018.11.032
7. Myatt L and Maloyan A. Obesity and placental function. Semin Reprod Med 2016; 34(01): 042-049. doi: 10.1055/s-0035-1570027
8. Arshad R, Karim N, Ara Hasan J. Effects of insulin on placental, fetal and maternal outcomes in gestational diabetes mellitus. *Pakistan Journal of Medical Sciences* 2014; 30(2): 240–244. doi.org/10.12669/pjms.302.4396
9. Lassance L, Miedl H, Absenger M, et al. Hyperinsulinemia stimulates angiogenesis of human fetoplacental endothelial cells: a possible role of insulin in placental hypervascularization in diabetes mellitus. *J Clin Endocrinol Metab* 2013; 98(9): E1438-E1447. doi:10.1210/jc.2013-1210
10. Cvitic S, Desoye G, Hiden U. Glucose, insulin, and oxygen interplay in placental hypervascularisation in diabetes mellitus. *Biomed Res Int* 2014; 2014: 145846. doi:10.1155/2014/145846
11. Sonagra AD, Biradar, SMKD, Murthy DSJ. Normal pregnancy- a state of insulin resistance. *Journal of clinical and Diagnostic Research* 2014; 8(11): CC01–CC3. doi.org/10.7860/JCDR/2014/10068.5081
12. Carr MC. The emergence of the metabolic syndrome with menopause. *J Clin Endocrinol Metab* 2003; 88(6): 2404-2411. doi:10.1210/jc.2003-030242

The evidence

Additional sources

Antioxidants, micronutrients, probiotics

Wesselink E, Koekkoek WAC, Grefte S, Witkamp RF, van Zanten ARH. Feeding mitochondria: Potential role of nutritional components to improve critical illness convalescence. *Clin Nutr* 2019; 38(3): 982-995. doi:10.1016/j.clnu.2018.08.032

Alzheimer's disease

Daulatzai MA. Cerebral hypoperfusion and glucose hypometabolism: Key pathophysiological modulators promote neurodegeneration, cognitive impairment, and Alzheimer's disease. *J Neurosci Res* 2017; 95(4): 943-972. doi: 10.1002/jnr.23777.

Krikorian R, Shidler MD, Dangelo K, Couch SC, Benoit SC, Clegg DJ. Dietary ketosis enhances memory in mild cognitive impairment. *Neurobiol Aging* 2012; 33(2): 425.e19–425.e27. doi: 10.1016/j.neurobiolaging.2010.10.006

Mosconi L, Pupi A, De Leon MJ. Brain glucose hypometabolism and oxidative stress in preclinical Alzheimer's disease. *Ann N Y Acad Sci* 2008; 1147: 180–195. doi:10.1196/annals.1427.007

Rhea EM, Banks WA. Role of the Blood-Brain Barrier in Central Nervous System Insulin Resistance. *Front Neurosci* 2019; 13: 521. doi: 10.3389/fnins.2019.00521

Stoykovich S, Gibas K. APOE ε4, the door to insulin-resistant dyslipidemia and brain fog? A case study. *Alzheimers Dement* 2019; 11: 264–269. doi: 10.1016/j.dadm.2019.01.009

Woods SC, Seeley RJ, Baskin DG, Schwartz MW. Insulin and the blood-brain barrier. *Curr Pharm Des* 2003; 9(10): 795-800.

Autonomic neuropathy

Diabetes.co.uk. Autonomic neuropathy. 15 January 2019. www.diabetes.co.uk/diabetes-complications/autonomic-neuropathy.html (accessed 28 June 2020)

Lee KO, Nam JS, Ahn CW, et al. Insulin resistance is independently associated with peripheral and autonomic neuropathy in Korean type 2 diabetic patients. *Acta Diabetol* 2012; 49: 97–103. doi.org/10.1007/s00592-010-0176-6

Bowel health, microbiome

Aron-Wisnewsky J, Clément K. The gut microbiome, diet, and links to cardiometabolic and chronic disorders. *Nat Rev Nephrol* 2016; 12(3): 169–181. doi:10.1038/nrneph.2015.191

Carabotti M, Scirocco A, Maselli M A, Severi C. The gut-brain axis: interactions between enteric microbiota, central and enteric nervous systems. *Ann Gastroenterol* 2015; 28(2): 203–209.

Clarke G, Stilling RM, Kennedy PJ, Stanton C, Cryan JF, Dinan TG. Minireview: Gut microbiota: the neglected endocrine organ. *Mol Endocrinol* 2014; 28(8): 1221-1238. doi: 10.1210/me.2014-1108.

Cryan JF, Dinan TG. Mind-altering microorganisms: the impact of the gut microbiota on brain and behaviour. *Nat Rev Neurosci* 2012; 13(10): 701-712. doi: 10.1038/nrn3346.

Diabetes.co.uk. Irritable bowel syndrome. 15 January 2019. www.diabetes.co.uk/conditions/irritable-bowel-syndrome-and-diabetes.html (accessed 30 June 2020)

Distrutti E, Monaldi L, Ricci P, Fiorucci S. Gut microbiota role in irritable bowel syndrome: New therapeutic strategies. *World Journal of Gastroenterology* 2016; 22(7): 2219–2241. doi.org/10.3748/wjg.v22.i7.2219

Franco-Obregon A, Gilbert JA. The Microbiome-Mitochondrion Connection: Common Ancestries, Common Mechanisms, Common Goals. *mSystems* 2017; 2(3): e00018-17. doi: 10.1128/mSystems.00018-17

Frasca G, Cardile V, Puglia C, et al. Gelatin tannate reduces the proinflammatory effects of lipopolysaccharide in human intestinal epithelial cells. *Clin Exp Gastroenterol* 2012; 5: 61–67. doi: 10.2147/CEG.S28792

Gagliardi A, Totino V, Cacciotti F, Iebba V, et al. Rebuilding the Gut Microbiota Ecosystem. *Int J Environ Res Public Health* 2018; 15(8): E1679. doi: 10.3390/ijerph15081679.

Gruber J, Kennedy BK. Microbiome and Longevity: Gut Microbes Send Signals to Host Mitochondria. *Cell* 2017; 169(7): 1168-1169. doi: 10.1016/j.cell.2017.05.048.

The evidence

Halfvarson J, Brislawn CJ, Lamendella R, et al. Dynamics of the human gut microbiome in inflammatory bowel disease. *Nat Microbiol* 2017; 2: 17004. doi:10.1038/nmicrobiol.2017.4

Han B, Sivaramakrishnan P, Lin C-CJ, Neve IAA, et al. Microbial Genetic Composition Tunes Host Longevity. *Cell* 2017; 169(7): 1249-1262.

Harvard Medical School. The gut-brain connection. Harvard Health Publishing. www.health.harvard.edu/diseases-and-conditions/the-gut-brain-connection (accessed 30 June 2020)

Karlsson FH, Tremaroli V, Nookaew I, et al. Gut metagenome in European women with normal, impaired and diabetic glucose control. *Nature* 2013; 498(7452): 99–103.

Kelly JR, Kennedy PJ, Cryan JF, Dinan TG, Clarke G, Hyland NP. Breaking down the barriers: the gut microbiome, intestinal permeability and stress-related psychiatric disorders. *Front Cell Neurosci* 2015; 9: 392. doi: 10.3389/fncel.2015.00392.

Kennedy PJ, Cryan JF, Dinan TG, Clarke G. Irritable bowel syndrome: a microbiome-gut-brain axis disorder? *World Journal of Gastroenterology* 2014; 20(39): 14105–14125. doi.org/10.3748/wjg.v20.i39.14105

Kirby TO, Ochoa-Reparaz J. The Gut Microbiome in Multiple Sclerosis: A Potential Therapeutic Avenue. *Medical Sciences* 2018; 6(3): 69.

Lawrence K, Hyde J. Microbiome restoration diet improves digestion, cognition and physical and emotional wellbeing. *PLoSOne* 2017; 12(6): e0179017.

Lernera A, Matthias B. Changes in intestinal tight junction permeability associated with industrial food additives explain the rising incidence of autoimmune disease. *Autoimmune Rev* 2015; 14(6): 479-489. doi:10.1016/j.autrev.2015.01.009

Lopetuso LR, Scaldaferri F, Bruno G, et al.The therapeutic management of gut barrier leaking: the emerging role for mucosal barrier protectors. *European Review for Medical and Pharmacological Sciences* 2015; 19(6): 1068-1076.

Maes M, Leunis JC. Normalization of leaky gut in chronic fatigue syndrome (CFS) is accompanied by a clinical improvement: effects of age, duration of illness and the translocation of LPS from gram-negative bacteria. *Neuro Endocrinol Lett* 2008; 29(6): 902-910.

Menni C, Zieter J, Pallister T, et al. Omega-3 fatty acids correlate with gut microbiome diversity and production of N-carbamylglutamate in middle aged and elderly women. *Scientific Reports* 2017; 7: 11079. doi: 10.1038/s41598-017-10382-2

Michielan A, D'Incà R. Intestinal Permeability in Inflammatory Bowel Disease: Pathogenesis, Clinical Evaluation, and Therapy of Leaky Gut. *Mediators of Inflammation* 2015: 628157. doi: 10.1155/2015/628157.

Mocking RJT, Harmsen I, Assies J, et al. Meta-analysis and meta-regression of omega-3 polyunsaturated fatty acid supplementation for major depressive disorder. *Translational Psychiatry* 2016; 6(3): e756. doi: 10.1038/tp.2016.29

Mokkala K, Röytiö H, Munukka E, Pietilä S, et al. Gut Microbiota Richness and Composition and Dietary Intake of Overweight Pregnant Women Are Related to Serum Zonulin Concentration, a Marker for Intestinal Permeability. *Journal of Nutrition* 2016; 146(9): 1694-1700. doi: 10.3945/jn.116.235358

Neuman H, Debelius JW, Knight R, Koren O. Microbial endocrinology: the interplay between the microbiota and the endocrine system. *FEMS Microbiol Rev* 2015; 39(4): 509-521. doi: 10.1093/femsre/fuu010.

O'Mahony SM, Clarke G, Borre YE, Dinan TG, Cryan JF. Serotonin, tryptophan metabolism and the brain-gut-microbiome axis. *Behav Brain Res* 2015; 277: 32–48. doi:10.1016/j.bbr.2014.07.027

Obrenovich MEM. Leaky gut, leaky brain? *Microorganisms* 2018; 6(4) pii: E107. doi: 10.3390/microorganisms6040107.

Pedersen HK, Gudmundsdottir V, Nielsen HB, et al. Human gut microbes impact host serum metabolome and insulin sensitivity. *Nature* 2016; 535(7612): 376–381,

Qin J, Li R, Raes J, et al. A human gut microbial gene catalogue established by metagenomic sequencing. *Nature* 2010; 464(7285): 59–65. doi: 10.1038/nature08821

Qinghui M, Kirby J, Reilly C, Xin M. Leaky Gut As a Danger Signal for Autoimmune Diseases. *Frontiers for Immunology* 2017; 8: 598

Robertson RC, Oriach S, Murphy K. Omega-3 polyunsaturated fatty acids critically regulate behaviour and gut microbiota development in adolescence and adulthood. *Brain Behav Immun* 2017; 59: 21-37. doi: 10.1016/j.jbi.2016.07.145.

Rooks MG, Garrett WS. Gut microbiota, metabolites and host immunity. *Nat Rev Immunol* 2016; 16(6): 341–352. doi:10.1038/nri.2016.42

Samsel A, Seneff S. Glyphosate, pathways to modern diseases II: Celiac sprue and gluten intolerance. *Interdiscip Toxicol* 2013; 6(4): 159–184. doi: 10.2478/intox-2013-0026

Scaldaferri F, Lopetuso LR, Petito V, et al. Gelatin tannate ameliorates acute colitis in mice by reinforcing mucus layer and modulating gut microbiota composition: Emerging role for 'gut barrier protectors' in IBD? *United European Gastroenterol J* 2014; 2(2): 113–122. doi: 10.1177/2050640614520867

Sender R, Fuchs S, Milo R. Revised Estimates for the Number of Human and Bacteria Cells in the Body. *PLoS Biology* 2016; 14(8): e1002533. doi.org/10.1371/journal.pbio.1002533

Sun MA, Rogers EW, Keating DJ. The Influence of the Gut Microbiome on Host Metabolism Through the Regulation of Gut Hormone Release. *Front Physiol* 2019; 10: 428. doi: 10.3389/fphys.2019.00428

Yano JM, Yu K, Donaldson GP, Shastri GG, et al. Indigenous bacteria from the gut microbiota regulate host serotonin biosynthesis. *Cell* 2015; 161(2): 264-276. doi: 10.1016/j.cell.2015.02.047.

Zeevi D, Korem T, Zmora N, et al. Personalized Nutrition by Prediction of Glycemic Responses. *Cell* 2015; 163(5): 1079–1094. doi:10.1016/j.cell.2015.11.001

Cancer

Denduluri SK, Idowu O, Wang Z et al. Insulin-like growth factor (IGF) signaling in tumorigenesis and the development of cancer drug resistance. *Genes & Diseases* 2015; 2(1): 13-25. doi.org/10.1016/j.gendis.2014.10.004

Fan X, Liu H, Liu M, et al. Increased utilization of fructose has a positive effect on the development of breast cancer. *Peer J* 2017; 5: e3804. doi: 10.7717/peerj.3804.

Friedrich N, Thuesen B, Jørgensen T, Juul A, Spielhagen C, Wallaschofksi H, Linneberg A. The association between IGF-I and insulin resistance: a general population study in Danish adults. *Diabetes Care* 2012; 35(4): 768–773. doi.org/10.2337/dc11-1833

Gillies RJ, Robey J, Gatenby RA).Causes and consequences of increased glucose metabolism of cancers. *J Nucl Med* 2008; 49(Suppl 2): 24S-42S. doi: 10.2967/jnumed.107.047258.

Khandekar MJ, Cohen P, Spiegelman BM. Molecular mechanisms of cancer development in obesity. *Nat Rev Cancer* 2011; 11(12): 886-895. doi:10.1038/nrc3174

Poff AM, Ari C, Arnold P, Seyfried TN, D'Agostino DP. Ketone supplementation decreases tumor cell viability and prolongs survival of mice with metastatic cancer. *Int J Cancer* 2014; 135(7): 1711–1720. doi: 10.1002/ijc.28809

Tsujimoto T, Kajio H, Sugiyama T. Association between hyperinsulinemia and increased risk of cancer death in nonobese and obese people: A population–based observational study. *Int J Cancer* 2017; 141(1): 102–111. doi: 10.1002/ijc.30729

Vasanti SM , Yanping L, Pan A, et al. Long-Term Consumption of Sugar-Sweetened and Artificially Sweetened Beverages and Risk of Mortality in US Adults. *Circulation* 2019; 139: 2113-2135. doi.org/10.1161/CIRCULATIONAHA.118.037401

Wanging Wen, Xiao Ou Shu, Honglan Li, et al. Dietary carbohydrates, fiber and breast cancer risk in Chinese women. *Am J Clin Nutr* 2009; 89(1): 283–289. doi: 10.3945/ajcn.2008.26356

Weber DD, Aminazdeh-Gohari S and Kofler B. Ketogenic diet in cancer therapy. *Aging* 2018: 10(2): 164-165

Weber DD, Aminzadeh-Gohari S, Tulipan J, et al. Ketogenic diet in the treatment of cancer – Where do we stand? *Molecular Metabolism* 2020; 33: 102-121. www.sciencedirect.com/science/article/pii/S2212877819304272

Chronic pain

Maloney EM, Boneva RS, Lin JM, Reeves WC. Chronic fatigue syndrome is associated with metabolic syndrome: results from a case-control study in Georgia. *Metabolism* 2010; 59(9): 1351-1357. doi: 10.1016/j.metabol.2009.12.019.

NHS England. Musculoskeletal conditions. www.england.nhs.uk/ourwork/clinical-policy/ltc/our-work-on-long-term-conditions/musculoskeletal/ (accessed 28 June 2020)

NHS England. Overview: Fibromyalgia. www.nhs.uk/conditions/

fibromyalgia/ (accessed 28 June 2020) www.nhs.uk/conditions/chronic-fatigue-syndrome-cfs/

Pyper D, Sutherland N, McInnes R, Barber S, Kennedy S. Recognition of fibromyalgia as a disability. *House of Commons Library* https://researchbriefings.parliament.uk/ResearchBriefing/Summary/CDP-2019-0003

Sluka KA, Clauw DJ. Neurobiology of fibromyalgia and chronic widespread pain. *Neuroscience* 2016; 338: 114-129. doi: 10.1016/j.neuroscience.2016.06.006.

Dental problems

Andriankaja OM, Munoz-Torrez F J, et al. Insulin resistance predicts the risk of gingival/periodontal inflammation. *Journal of Periodontology* 2018; 89(5): 549-557.

Song, I-S, Han, K, Park Y-M et al. Severe Periodontitis Is Associated with Insulin Resistance in Non-abdominal Obese Adults. *The Journal of Clinical Endocrinology & Metabolism* 2016; 11: 4251-4259. doi.org/10.1210/jc.2016-2061

Verhulst, M J L, Loos, B G, Gerdes, V E A and Teeuw, W J. Evaluating All Potential Oral Complications of Diabetes Mellitus. *Frontiers in Endocrinology* 18 February 2019. doi.org/10.3389/fendo.2019.00056

Diabetes, type 2

Athinarayanan SJ, Adams RN, Hallberg SJ, McKenzie AL, Bhanpuri NH, Campbell WW, Volek JS. Long-term Effects of a Novel Continuous Remote Care Intervention Including Nutritional Ketosis for the Management of Type 2 Diabetes: A 2-Year Non-randomized Clinical Trial. *Frontiers in Endocrinology* 2019; 10: 348. doi: 10.3389/fendo.2019.00348.

Diabetes.co.uk. The liver and blood glucose levels. 15 January 2019. www.diabetes.co.uk/body/liver-and-blood-glucose-levels.html (accessed 29 June 2020)

Hattling M, Tavares CDJ, Sharabi K, RInes AK, Puigserver P. Insulin regulation of gluconeogenesis. *Ann N Y Acad Sci* 2018; 1411(1): 21–35. doi: 10.1111/nyas.13435

Sainsbury E, Kizirian NV, Partridge SR, Gill T, Colagiuri S, Gibson AA. Effect of dietary carbohydrate restriction on glycemic control in adults with diabetes: A systematic review and meta-analysis. *Diabetes Res Clin Pract* 2018; 139: 239-252. doi: 10.1016/j.diabres.2018.02.026.

Snorgaard O, Poulsen GM, Andersen HK, Astrup A. Systematic review and meta-analysis of dietary carbohydrate restriction in patients with type 2 diabetes. *BMJ Open Diabetes Research and Care* 2017; 5: e000354. doi: 10.1136/bmjdrc-2016-000354

Turton J, Brinkworth GD, Field R, Parker H, Rooney. An evidence-based approach to developing low-carbohydrate diets for type 2 diabetes management: A systematic review of interventions and methods. *Diabetes Obes Metab* 2019; 21(11): 2513-2525. doi: 10.1111/dom.13837.

Unwin D. Low carbohydrate diet to achieve weight loss and improve HbA1c in type 2 diabetes and prediabetes: experience from one general practice. *Practical Diabetes* 2014; 31(2): 76-79. www.practicaldiabetes.com/wp-content/uploads/sites/29/2016/03/Low-carbohydrate-diet-to-achieve-weight-loss-and-improve-HbA1c-in-type-2-diabetes-and-pre-diabetes-experience-from-one-general-practice.pdf

Volek JS, Feinman RD. Carbohydrate restriction improves the features of Metabolic Syndrome. Metabolic Syndrome may be defined by the response to carbohydrate restriction. *Nutr Metab* 2005; 2: 31.

Wang LL, Wang, Q, Hong, Y, Ojo, O, JIang, Q, Hou YY, Huang YH, Wang XH. The Effect of Low-Carbohydrate Diet on Glycemic Control in Patients with Type 2 Diabetes Mellitus. *Nutrients* 2018; 10(6). pii: E661. doi: 10.3390/nu10060661

Dietary fat and fatty acids

Angerer P, von Schacky C. n-3 polyunsaturated fatty acids and the cardiovascular system. *Curr Opin Lipidol* 2000; 11(1): 57-63.

BBC 2: Trust Me I'm a Doctor. Which oils are best to cook with? www.bbc.co.uk/programmes/articles/3t902pqt3C7nGN99hVRFc1y/which-oils-are-best-to-cook-with (29 June 2020)

Berbert AA, Kondo CR, Almendra CL, et al. Supplementation of fish oil and olive oil in patients with rheumatoid arthritis. *Nutrition* 2005; 21: 131-136.

Calder PC. n-3 polyunsaturated fatty acids, inflammation, and inflammatory diseases. *Am J Clin Nutr* 2006; 83(6 Suppl): 1505S-1519S. doi: 10.1093/ajcn/83.6.1505S.

Dalleau S, Baradat M, Gueraud F, Huc L. Cell death and diseases related to oxidative stress:4-hydroxynonenal (HNE) in the balance. *Cell Death Differ* 2013; 20(12): 1615–1630. doi: 10.1038/cdd.2013.138

Derbyshire E. Brain Health across the Lifespan: A Systematic Review on the Role of Omega-3 Fatty Acid Supplements. *Nutrients* 2018; 10(8): 1094. doi: 10.3390/nu10081094

Goldberg RJ, Katz J. A meta-analysis of the analgesic effects of omega-3 polyunsaturated fatty acid sup-plementation for inflammatory joint pain. *Pain* 2007; 129(1-2): 210-223. doi: 10.1016/j.pain.2007.01.020

Innes JK, Calder PC. The Differential Effects of Eicosapentaenoic Acid and Docosahexaenoic Acid on Cardiometabolic Risk Factors: A Systematic Review. *Int J Mol Sci* 2018; 19(2): E532. doi: 10.3390/ijms19020532.

Khanapure SP, Garvey D S, Janero DR, Letts LG. Eicosanoids in inflammation: biosynthesis, pharmacology, and therapeutic frontiers. *Curr Top Med Chem* 2007; 7(3): 311-340.

Kris-Etherton PM, Shaffe-Taylor D, Yu-Poth S, at al. Polyunsaturated fatty acids in the food chain in the United States. *American Journal of Clinical Nutrition* 2000; 71(1): 179S–188S. doi.org/10.1093/ajcn/71.1.179S

Mori TA. Omega-3 fatty acids and blood pressure. *Cell Mol Biol* 2010; 56(1): 83-92.

Song J, Park J, Jung J, et al. Analysis of Trans Fat in Edible Oils with Cooking Process. *Toxicol Res* 2015; 31(3): 307-312. doi:10.5487/TR.2015.31.3.307

Teng KT, Voon PT, Cheng HM, Nesaretnam K. Effects of partially hydrogenated, semi-saturated, and high oleate vegetable oils on inflammatory markers and lipids. *Lipids* 2010; 45(5): 385-392. doi: 10.1007/s11745-010-3416-1.

Dietary sugar advice and recommendations

World Health Organization. WHO calls on countries to to reduce sugars intake among adults and children. 4 March 2015. www.who.int/mediacentre/news/releases/2015/sugar-guideline/en/ (accessed 29 June 2020) (WHO recommendation, sugar (6 teaspoons))

Exercise

Bird SR, Hawley JA. Update on the effects of physical activity on insulin sensitivity in humans. *BMJ Open Sport Exerc Med* 2016; 2(1): e000143. doi: 10.1136/bmjsem-2016-000143

Carter HN, Chen CCW, Hood DA. Mitochondria, Muscle Health, and Exercise with Advancing Age. *Physiology* 2015; 30(3): 208-223. doi.org/10.1152/physiol.00039.2014

Cook NJ, Ng A, Read GF, Harris B, Riad-Fahmy D. Salivary cortisol for monitoring adrenal activity during marathon runs. *Horm Res* 1987; 25(1): 18–23. doi:10.1159/000180628

Dirks ML, Wall BT, van de Valk B, et al. One week of bed rest leads to substantial muscle atrophy and induces whole-body insulin resistance in the absence of skeletal muscle lipid accumulation. *Diab* 2016; 65(10): 2862–2875.

Flynn MG, McFarlin BK, Markofski MM. The Anti-Inflammatory Actions of Exercise Training. *American Journal of Lifestyle Medicine* 2007; 1(3): 220–235. doi.org/10.1177/1559827607300283

Fry RW, Grove JR, Morton AR, Zeroni PM, Gaudieri S, Keast D. (1994). Psychological and immunological correlates of acute overtraining. *British Journal of Sports Medicine* 1994; 28(4): 241–246. doi.org/10.1136/bjsm.28.4.241

Gougeon R. Insulin resistance of protein metabolism in type 2 diabetes and impact on dietary needs: a review. *Can J Diabetes* 2013; 37(2): 115–120. doi:10.1016/j.jcjd.2013.01.007

Hakkinen K, Pakarinen A. Acute hormonal responses to two different fatiguing heavy-resistance protocols in male athletes. *Journal of Applied Physiology* 1993; 74(2): 882-887. doi.org/10.1152/jappl.1993.74.2.882

Macpherson H, Teo W-P, Schneider LA, Smith AE. A life-long

approach to physical activity for brain health. *Frontiers in Aging Neuroscience* 2017; 9(147): 1-12.

McCray CJ, Agarwal SK. Stress and autoimmunity. *Immunol Allergy Clin North Am* 2011; 31(1): 1–18. doi:10.1016/j.iac.2010.09.004

Oliver AN, Hood DA. Exercise is mitochondrial medicine for muscle. *Sports Medicine and Health Science* 2019; 1(1): 11-18. doi.org/10.1016/j.smhs.2019.08.008

Young SN. How to increase serotonin in the human brain without drugs. *Journal of Psychiatry and Neuroscience* 2007; 32(6): 394–399.

Fatty liver

Albillos A, Lario M, Alvarez-Mon M.Cirrhosis-associated immune dysfunction:Distinctive features and clinical relevance. *Journal of Hepatology* 2014; 61(6): 1385-1396. doi.org/10.1016/j.jhep.2014.08.010

Byrne CDH. Dorothy Hodgkin Lecture 2012: Non-alcoholic fatty liver disease, insulin resistance and ectopic fat: a new problem in diabetes management. *Diabetic Medicine* 2012; 29(9): 1098-1107. doi: 10.1111/j.1464-5491.2012.03732.x

Campo L, Eiseler S, Apfel T, Pyrsopoulos N. Fatty Liver Disease and Gut Microbiota: A Comprehensive Update. *J Clin Transl Hepatol* 2019; 7(1): 56-60. doi:10.14218/JCTH.2018.00008

Carr RM, Correnti J. Insulin resistance in clinical and experimental alcoholic liver disease. *Annals of the New York Academy of Science* 2015; 1353(1): 1-20. doi: 10.1111/nyas.12787

Cederbaum AI. Alcohol metabolism. *Clin Liver Dis* 2012; 16(4): 667–685. doi: 10.1016/j.cld.2012.08.002

Kim JI, Lee DY, Lee YJ, Park KJ, Kim KH, Kim JW, Kim W-H. Chronic alcohol consumption potentiates the development of diabetes through pancreatic β-cell dysfunction. *World J Biol Chem* 2015; 6(1): 1–15.

Kubes P, Jenne C. Immune responses in the liver. *Annual Review of Immunology* 2018; 36: 247-277. doi.org/10.1146/annurev-immunol-051116-052415

Lustig RH. Fructose: It's 'Alcohol Without the Buzz'. *Adv Nutr* 2013; 4(2): 226–235. doi: 10.3945/an.112.002998

Mohamed J, Nafizah AHN, et al. Mechanisms of Diabetes-Induced

Liver Damage: The role of oxidative stress and inflammation. *Sultan Qaboos Univ Med J* 2016; 16(2): e132–e141

Taipale T, Seppälä I, Raitoharju E, et al. Fatty liver is associated with blood pathways of inflammatory response, immune system activation and prothrombotic state in Young Finns Study. *Sci Rep* 2018; 8: 10358. doi.org/10.1038/s41598-018-28563-y

Ter Horst KW, Serlie MJ. Fructose Consumption, Lipogenesis, and Non-Alcoholic Fatty Liver Disease. *Nutrients* 2017; 9(9): 981. doi:10.3390/nu9090981

Fruit, berries and vegetables

Mazzoni L, Perez-Lopez P, Giampieri F, et al. The genetic aspects of berries: from field to health. *J Sci Food Agric* 2016; 96(2): 365-71. doi: 10.1002/jsfa.7216.

Skrovankova S, Sumczynski D, Mlcek J, et al. Bioactive Compounds and Antioxidant Activity in Different Types of Berries. *Int J Mol Sci* 2015; 16(10): 24673-2706. doi: 10.3390/ijms161024673.

Wolfe KL, Kang X, He X, et al. Cellular Antioxidant Activity of Common Fruits. *J Agric Food Chem* 2008; 56(18): 8418-8426.

Glaucoma and retinal degeneration

Tirsi A, Bruehl H, Sweat V et al. Retinal Vessel Abnormalities are associated with Elevated Fasting Insulin Levels and Cerebral Atrophy in Non-Diabetic Individuals. *Ophthalmology* 2009; 116(6): 1175–1181. doi: 10.1016/j.ophtha.2008.12.046

Wong-Riley MT. Energy metabolism of the visual system. *Eye and Brain* 2010; 2: 99–116. doi.org/10.2147/EB.S9078

Gout

Arthritis Foundation. Fructose and gout. *Arthritis Today Magazine*. 15 February 2020. http://blog.arthritis.org/gout/fructose-sugar-gout/ (accessed 30 June 2020)

Barskova VG, Eliseev MS, Nasonov EL, Iakunina IA, Zilov AV, Il'inykh EV. Insulin resistance syndrome in patients with gout and its influence on formation of clinical characteristics of the disease. *Ter Arkh* 2004; 76(5): 51-56.

Choi HK. Prevalence of the Metabolic Syndrome in Individuals with Hyperuricemia. *American Journal of Medicine* 2007; 120(5): 442–447.

Juraschek SP, McAdams-Demarco M, Gelber AC, et al. Effects of Lowering Glycemic Index of Dietary Carbohydrate on Plasma Uric Acid Levels: The OmniCarb Randomized Clinical Trial. *Arthritis Rheumatol* 2016; 68(5): 1281-1289. doi:10.1002/art.39527

Neogi T, Chen C, Niu J, Chaisson C, Hunter DJ, Zhang Y. Alcohol quantity and type on risk of recurrent gout attacks: an internet-based case-crossover study. *Am J Med* 2014; 127(4): 311-318. doi:10.1016/j.amjmed.2013.12.019

Grains and fibre

Fasano A, Sapone A, Zevallos V, Schuppan D. Nonceliac gluten sensitivity. *Gastroenterology* 2015; 148(6): 1195-1204. doi: 10.1053/j.gastro.2014.12.049.

De Punder K, Pruimboom L. The Dietary Intake of Wheat and other Cereal Grains and Their Role in Inflammation. *Nutrients* 2013; 5(3): 771-787.

McGuirk A. Carbohydrates, fibre and a healthy diet (letter). *Guardian* 15 Jan 2019. www.theguardian.com/society/2019/jan/15/carbohydrates-fibre-and-a-healthy-diet

Molina-Infante J, Santolaria S, Sanders DS, Fernández-Bañares F. Systematic review: noncoeliac gluten sensitivity. *Aliment Pharmacol Ther* 2015; 41(9): 807-820. doi: 10.1111/apt.13155.

Sanz Y, De Pama G, Laparra M. Unraveling the ties between celiac disease and intestinal microbiota. *Int Rev Immunol* 2011; 30(4): 207-218. doi: 10.3109/08830185.2011.599084.

Tovoli F, Masi C, Guidetti E, Negrini G, Paterini P, Bolondi L. Clinical and diagnostic aspects of gluten related disorders. *World J Clin Cases* 2015; 3(3): 275-284. doi: 10.12998/wjcc.v3.i3.275.

Heart disease and cholesterol

Attia P. The straight dope on cholesterol – Part V. Peter Attia MD. 23 May 2012. https://peterattiamd.com/the-straight-dope-on-cholesterol-part-v/ (accessed 4 July 2020)

Aubert G, Martin OJ, Horton JL, et al. The Failing Heart Relies on Ketone Bodies as a Fuel [published correction appears in Circulation. 2018 Oct 9;138(15):e422]. *Circulation* 2016; 133(8): 698-705. doi:10.1161/CIRCULATIONAHA.115.017355

Ho KL, Zhang L, Wagg C, Batran RA, et al. Increased ketone body oxidation provides additional energy for the failing heart without improving cardiac efficiency. *Cardiovascular Research* 2019; 115(11): 1606-1616. doi: 10.1093/cvr/cvz045.

Manifold-Wheeler BC, Elmore BO, Triplett KD, Castleman MJ, Otto M, Hall PR. Serum Lipoproteins Are Critical for Pulmonary Innate Defense against Staphylococcus aureus Quorum Sensing. *J Immunol* 2016; 196(1): 328-335. doi:10.4049/jimmunol.1501835

Mason P. Dr Paul Mason talk: High cholesterol on a ketogenic diet – 2019 update. www.youtube.com/watch?v=TRB0jOfymLk

Packard C, Caslake M, Shepherd J. The role of small, dense low density lipoprotein (LDL): a new look. *International Journal of Cardiology* 2000; 74(1): S17-S22.

Ramachandran R, Wierzbicki AS. Statins, Muscle Disease and Mitochondria. *Journal of Clinical Medicine* 2017: 6(8): 75.

Ravnskov U, Diamond DM, Hama R, Hamazaki T, et al. Lack of an Association or an inverse Association between low-sdensity-lipoprotein cholesterol and mortality in the elderly: a systematic review. *BMJ Open* 2016; 6(6): e010401.
doi: 10.1136/bmjopen-2015-010401.

van Peet PG, Drewes YM, de Craen AJ, Westendorp RG, Gussekloo J, de Ruijter W. Prognostic value of cardiovascular disease status: the Leiden 85-plus study. *Age* 2013; 35(4): 1433-1444. doi:10.1007/s11357-012-9443-5

Wood RJ, Volek JS, Liu Y, et al. Carbohydrate Restriction Alters Lipoprotein Metabolism by Modifying VLDL, LDL, and HDL Subfraction Distribution and Size in Overweight Men. *Journal of Nutrition* 2006; 136(2): 384–389. doi.org/10.1093/jn/136.2.384

World Health Organization. Cardiovascular diseases. www.who.int/health-topics/cardiovascular-diseases (accessed 4 July 2020)

Zampelas A, Magriplis E. New Insights into Cholesterol Functions: A Friend or an Enemy? *Nutrients* 2019; 11(7): 1645.
doi: 10.3390/nu11071645

Immunity

Clemente-Casares X, Zhou AC, Watts TH, et al. Insulin Receptor-Mediated Stimulation Boosts T Cell Immunity during Inflammation and Infection. *Cell Metabolism* 2018; 28(6): 922-934.

Fernandez-Real JM, Pickup JC. Innate immunity, insulin resistance and type 2 diabetes. *Trends Endocrinol Metab* 2008; 19(1): 10-16.

Finucane FM, Davenport C. Coronavirus and Obesity. Could Insulin Resistance Mediate the Severity of Covid-19 Infection? *Front Public Health* 12 May 2020. doi.org/10.3389/fpubh.2020.00184

Ieronymaki E, Daskalaki MG, Lyroni K, Tsatsanis C. Insulin Signaling and Insulin Resistance Facilitate Trained Immunity in Macrophages Through Metabolic and Epigenetic Changes. *Front Immunol* 12 June 2019. doi.org/10.3389/fimmu.2019.01330

Winer DA, Luck H, Tsai S, Winer S. The Intestinal Immune System in Obesity and Insulin Resistance. *Cell Metabolism* 2016; 23(3): 413-426.

Inflammation

Aeberli I, Gerber PA, Hochuli M, et al. Low to moderate sugar-sweetened beverage consumption impairs glucose and lipid metabolism and promotes inflammation in healthy young men: a randomized controlled trial. *Am J Clin Nutr* 2011; 94(2): 479-485. doi: 10.3945/ajcn.111.013540.

Bajwa E, Pointer CB, Klegeris A. The Role of Mitochondrial Damage-Associated Molecular Patterns in Chronic Neuroinflammation. *Mediators of Inflammation* 2019; 2019: Article ID 4050796. doi.org/10.1155/2019/4050796

de Luca C, Olefsky JM. Inflammation and Insulin Resistance. FEBS Lett. Author manuscript; available in PMC 2009 Jan 9. *FEBS Letters* 2008; 582(1): 97–105. doi: 10.1016/j.febslet.2007.11.057

Rehman K, Akash MSH. Mechanisms of inflammatory responses and development of insulin resistance: how are they interlinked? *Journal of Biomedical Science* 2016; 23: article no 87.

Ricciotti E, Fitzgerald GA. Prostaglandins and Inflammation. *Arterioscler Thromb Vasc Biol* 2011; 31(5): 986-1000. doi: 10.1161/ATVBAHA.110.207449.

Shimobayashi M, Albert V, Woelnerhanssen B, et al. Insulin resistance causes inflammation in adipose tissue. 2018. *J Clin Invest* 2018; 128(4): 1538–1550. doi: 10.1172/JCI96139

Inner ear problems

Albernaz PL. Hearing Loss, Dizziness and Carbohydrate Metabolism. *International Archives of Otorhinolaryngology* 2016; 20(3); 261-270.

D'Avila C, Lavinsky L. Glucose and insulin profiles and their correlations in Meniere's disease. *Int Tinnitus J* 2005; 11(2): 170-176.

Lavinsky L, Oliveira MW, Bassanesi HJ, D'Avila C, Lavinsky M. Hyperinsulinemia and tinnitus: a historical cohort. *Int Tinnitus J* 2004; 10(1): 24-30.

Mangabeira Albernaz PL. Hearing Loss, Dizziness, and Carbohydrate Metabolism. *International Archives of Otorhinolaryngology* 2016; 20(3): 261-270.

Webster G, Sens PM, Salmito MC, et al. Hyperinsulinemia and hyperglycaemia:risk factors for recurrence of benign paroxysmal positional vertigo. *Braz J Otorhinolaryngol* 2015; 81(4): 347-51. doi: 10.1016/j.bjorl.2014.09.008.

Low-carb diet

Accurso A, Bernstein RK, Dahlqvist A, et al. Dietary carbohydrate restriction in type 2 diabetes mellitus and metabolic syndrome: Time for a critical appraisal. *Nutr Metab* 2008; 5: 9. doi.org/10.1186/1743-7075-5-9

Athinarayanan SJ, Adams RN, Hallberg SJ, McKenzie AL, et al. Long-term effects of a novel continuous remote care intervention including nutritional ketosis for the management of type 2 diages: a 2-year non-randomized clinical trial. *Front Endocrinol* 5 June 2019. doi.org/10.3389/fendo.2019.00348

Bae HR, Kim DH, Park MH, et al. β-Hydroxybutyrate suppresses inflammasome formation by ameliorating endoplasmic reticulum stress via AMPK activation. *Oncotarget* 2016; 7(41): 66444–66454. doi: 10.18632/oncotarget.12119

Castro AI, Gomez-Arbelaez D, Crujeiras AB, et al. Effect of A Very Low-Calorie Ketogenic Diet on Food and Alcohol Cravings,

Physical and Sexual Activity, Sleep Disturbances, and Quality of Life in Obese Patients. *Nutrients* 2018; 10(10): 1348. doi: 10.3390/nu10101348

Cunnane SC, Courchesne-Loyer A, St-Pierre V, et al. Can Ketones Compensate for Deteriorating Brain Glucose Uptake During Aging? Implications for the Risk and Treatment of Alzheimer's Disease. *Ann N Y Acad Sci* 2016; 1367(1): 12–20. doi:10.1111/nyas.12999

Diabetes.co.uk. Low-carb diet side effects. 15 January 2019. www.diabetes.co.uk/diet/low-carb-diet-side-effects.html (accessed 30 June 2020)

Feinman RD, Pogozelski WK, Astrup A, et al. Dietary carbohydrate restriction as the first approach in diabetes management: Critical review and evidence base. *Nutrition* 2015; 31(1): 1–13. doi.org/10.1016/j.nut.2014.06.011

Forsythe CE, Phinney SD, Fernanzed ML, et al. Comparison of low fat and low carbohydrate diets on circulating fatty acid composition and markers of inflammation. *Lipids* 2008; 43(1): 65-77.

Gasior M, Rogawski MA, Hartman AL. Neuroprotective and disease-modifying effects of the ketogenic diet. *Behav Pharmacol* 2006; 17(5-6): 431–439.

Gjuladin-Hellon T, Davies IG, Penson P, Baghbadorani R. Effects of carbohydrate-restricted diets on low-density lipoprotein cholesterol levels in overweight and obese adults: a systematic review and meta-analysis. *Nutr Rev* 2019; 77(3): 161-180. doi: 10.1093/nutrit/nuy049.

Hallböök T, Lundgren J, Rosén I. Ketogenic diet improves sleep quality in children with therapy-resistant epilepsy. *Epilepsia* 2007; 48(1): 59-65.

Huntriss R, Campbell M, Bedwell C. The interpretation and effect of a low-carbohydrate diet in the management of type 2 diabetes: a systematic review and meta-analysis of randomised controlled trials. *Eur J Clin Nutr* 2018; 72(3): 311-325. doi: 10.1038/s41430-017-0019-4.

Krikorian R, Shidler MD, Dangelo K, et al. Dietary ketosis enhances memory in mild cognitive impairment. *Neurobiol Aging* 2012; 33(2): 425.e19–425.e27. doi: 10.1016/j.neurobiolaging.2010.10.006

Mansoor N, Vinknes KJ, Veierød MB, Retterstøl K. Effects of

low-carbohydrate diets v. low-fat diets on body weight and cardiovascular risk factors: a meta-analysis of randomised controlled trials. *Br J Nutr* 2016; 115(3): 466-479. doi: 10.1017/S0007114515004699.

McCarthy MF, DiNicolantonio JJ, O'Keefe JH. Ketosis may promote brain macroautophagy by activating Sirt1 and hypoxia-inducible factor-1. *Med Hypotheses* 2015; 85(5): 631-639. doi: 10.1016/j.mehy.2015.08.002.

McClernon FJ, Yancy WS Jr, Eberstein JA, Atkins RC, Westman EC. The effects of a low-carbohydrate ketogenic diet and a low-fat diet on mood, hunger, and other self-reported symptoms. *Obesity* 2007; 15(1): 182-187.

Sackner-Bernstein J, Kanter D, Kaul S. Dietary Intervention for Overweight and Obese Adults: Comparison of Low-Carbohydrate and Low-Fat Diets. A Meta-Analysis. *PLoS One* 2015; 10(10): e0139817. doi: 10.1371/journal.pone.0139817.

Sainsbury E, Kizirian NV, Partridge SR, Gill T, Colagiuri S, Gibson AA. Effect of dietary carbohydrate restriction on glycemic control in adults with diabetes: A systematic review and meta-analysis. *Diabetes Res Clin Pract* 2018; 139: 239-252. doi: 10.1016/j.diabres.2018.02.026.

Snorgaard O, Poulsen GM, Andersen HK, Astrup A. Systematic review and meta-analysis of dietary carbohydrate restriction in patients with type 2 diabetes. *BMJ Open Diabetes Res Care* 2017 23; 5(1): e000354. doi: 10.1136/bmjdrc-2016-000354.

Turton J, Brinkworth GD, Field R, Parker H, Rooney K. An evidence-based approach to developing low-carbohydrate diets for type 2 diabetes management: A systematic review of interventions and methods. *Diabetes Obes Metab* 2019; 21(11): 2513-2525. doi: 10.1111/dom.13837.

Volek JS, Fernandez ML, Feinman RD, Phinney SD. Dietary carbohydrate restriction induces a unique metabolic state positively affecting atherogenic dyslipidemia, fatty acid partitioning, and metabolic syndrome. *Prog Lipid Res* 2008; 47(5): 307-318. doi:10.1016/j.plipres.2008.02.003

Westman EC, Feinman RD, Mavropoulos JC, et al. Low-carbohydrate nutrition and metabolism. *Am J Clin Nutr* 2007; 86(2): 276–284.

Yancy WS, Foy M, Chalecki AM, Vernon MC, Westman EC. A low-carbohydrate, ketogenic diet to treat type 2 diabetes. *Nutr Metab* 2005; 2: 34.

Mental health

Brown D, Triggle N. Mental health: 10 charts on the scale of the problem. BBC News: Health. 4 December 2018. www.bbc.co.uk/news/health-41125009 (accessed 30 June 2020)

Kullmann S, Heni M, Hallschmid M, Fritsche A. Brain Insulin Resistance at the Crossroads of Metabolic and Cognitive Disorders in Humans. *Physiological Reviews* 3 August 2016. www.physiology.org/doi/full/10.1152/physrev.00032.2015?url_ver=Z39.88-2003&rfr_id=ori%3Arid%3Acrossref.org&rfr_dat=cr_pub%3Dpubmed&

Mind. Mental health facts and statistics. www.mind.org.uk/information-support/types-of-mental-health-problems/statistics-and-facts-about-mental-health/how-common-are-mental-health-problems/#.Xh_9pC2ca1s (accessed 30 June 2020)

Steele CB, Thomas CC, Henley SJ, Massetti GM, et al. Vital signs: trends in incidence of cancers associated with overweight and obesity – United States, 2005-2014. Centers for Disease Control and Prevention: *Morbidity and Mortality Weekly Report (MMWR)* 2017; 66(39): 1052-1058. www.cdc.gov/mmwr/volumes/66/wr/mm6639e1.htm?s_cid=mm6639e1_ehttps://www.who.int/news-room/fact-sheets/detail/depression

World Health Organization. Depression. www.who.int/health-topics/depression#tab=tab_1 (accessed 3 July 2020)

World Health Organization. Depression. Key Facts. 30 January 2020. www.who.int/news-room/fact-sheets/detail/depression (accessed 3 July 2020)

Yan YX, Xiao HB, Wang SS, et al. Investigation of the Relationship Between Chronic Stress and Insulin Resistance in a Chinese Population. *J Epidemiol* 2016; 26(7): 355-360. doi:10.2188/jea.JE20150183

Young SE, Mainous AG 3rd, Carnemolla M. Hyperinsulinemia and cognitive decline in a middle-aged cohort. *Diabetes Care* 2006; 29(12): 2688-2693. doi:10.2337/dc06-0915

Mitochondria

Andrade MJ, Jayaprakash C, Bhat S, et al. Antibiotics-Induced Obesity: A Mitochondrial Perspective. *Public Health Genomics* 2017; 20: 257–273.

Cox P, et al. Nutritional Ketosis Alters Fuel Preference and Thereby Endurance Performance in Athletes. *Cell Metabolism* 2016; 24: 256-268.

de Almeida Chuffa LG, Seiva FRF, Cucielo MS, et al. Cellular and Molecular Life Sciences 2019; 76: 837-863. doi.org/10.1007/s00018-018-2963-0

Kanasaki K, Kawakita E, Koya D. Relevance of Autophagy Induction by Gastrointestinal Hormones: Focus on the Incretin-Based Drug Target and Glucagon. *Front Pharmacol* 16 May 2019. doi.org/10.3389/fphar.2019.00476

Kim JA, Wei Y, Sowers JR. Role of mitochondrial dysfunction in insulin resistance. *Circulation Research* 2008; 102(4): 401–414. doi.org/10.1161/CIRCRESAHA.107.165472

Kumar A, Singh A. A review on mitochondrial restorative mechanism of antioxidants in Alzheimer's disease and other neurological conditions. *Frontiers in Pharmacology* 2015; 6: 206. doi: 10.3389/fphar.2015.00206. eCollection 2015.

Mills EL, Kelly B, Logan A, et al. Succinate Dehydrogenase Supports Metabolic Repurposing of Mitochondria to Drive Inflammatory Macrophages. *Cell* 2016; 167(2): 457-470.e13. doi:10.1016/j.cell.2016.08.064

Nicolson GL. Mitochondrial dysfunction and chronic disease: treatment with natural supplements. *Alternative Therapies in Health and Medicine* 2014r;20 Suppl 1:18-25.

Parker BA, Walton CM, Carr ST, et al. β-Hydroxybutyrate Elicits Favorable Mitochondrial Changes in Skeletal Muscle. *Int J Mol Sci* 2018; 19(8): 2247. doi:10.3390/ijms19082247

Serrano JCE, Cassanye A, Martín-Gari M, Granado-Serrano AB, Portero-Otín M. Effect of Dietary Bioactive Compounds on Mitochondrial and Metabolic Flexibility. *Diseases* 2016;10 4(1): pii: E14. doi: 10.3390/diseases4010014.

Seyfried TN. Cancer as a mitochondrial metabolic disease. *Frontiers in Cell and Developmental Biology* 2015; 3: 43.

Sullivan EM, Pennington ER, Green WD, Bet al. Mechanisms by Which Dietary Fat ty Acids Regulate Mitochondrial Structure-Function in Health and Disease. *Advances in Nutrition* 2018; 9(3): 247-262.

Takahashi M, Takahashi K. Water-soluble CoQ10 as A Promising Anti-aging Agent for Neurological Dysfunction in Brain Mitochondria. *Antioxidants* 2019; 11; 8(3): pii: E61.

Weinberg SE,, Sena LA, Chandel NS. Mitochondria in the regulation of innate and adaptive immunity. *Immunity* 2015; 42(3): 406–417. doi.org/10.1016/j.immuni.2015.02.002

Wesselink E, Koekkoek WAC, Grefte S, Witkamp RF, van Zanten ARH. Feeding mitochondria: Potential role of nutritional components to improve critical illness convalescence. *Clinical Nutrition* 2018 Aug 31. pii: S0261-5614(18)32426-9.

Muscle mass

Guillet C, Boirie Y. Insulin resistance: a contributing factor to age-related muscle mass loss? *Diabetes Metabolism* 2005; 31(1): 5S20-5S26. doi.org/10.1016/S1262-3636(05)73648-X

Ostler JE, Maurya SK, Dials J, et al. Effects of insulin resistance on skeletal muscle growth and exercise capacity in type 2 diabetic mouse models. *Am J Physiol Endocrinol Metab* 2014; 306(6): E592-E605. doi:10.1152/ajpendo.00277.2013

Obesity

Foster GD, Wyatt Hill JO, Makris AP, Rosenbaum DL, et al. Weight and Metabolic Outcomes After 2 Years on a Low-Carbohydrate Versus Low-Fat Diet. *Ann Intern Med* 2010; 153(3): 147–157. doi: 10.1059/0003-4819-153-3-201008030-00005

Hashimoto Y, Fukuda T, Oyabu C, Tanaka M, Asano M, Yamazaki M, Fukui M. Impact of low-carbohydrate diet on body composition: meta-analysis of randomized controlled studies. *Obes Rev* 2016; 17(6): 499-509. doi: 10.1111/obr.12405. Epub 2016 Apr 5.

Laforest S, Labrecque J, Michaud A, Cianflone K, Tchernof A. Adipocyte size as a determinant of metabolic disease and adipose tissue dysfunction. *Crit Rev Clin Lab Sci* 2015; 52(6): 301-13. doi: 10.3109/10408363.2015.1041582.

Ludwig DS, Majzoub JA, Al-Zahrani A, Dallas GE et al. High glycemic index foods, overeating, and obesi-ty. *Pediatrics* 1999; 103(3): E26.

Mansoor N, Vinknes KJ, Veierod MB, Retterstol K. Effects of low-carbohydrate diets v. low-fat diets on body weight and cardiovascular risk factors: a meta-analysis of randomised controlled trials. *Br J Nutr* 2016; 115(3): 466-479. doi: 10.1017/S0007114515004699.

Noakes TD. So What Comes First: The Obesity or the Insulin Resistance? And Which Is More Important? *Clinical Chemistry* 2020; 64(1): 7–9. doi.org/10.1373/clinchem.2017.282962

Sackner-Bernstein J, Kanter D, Kaul S. Dietary Intervention for Overweight and Obese Adults: Comparison of Low-Carbohydrate and Low-Fat Diets. A meta-analysis. *PLoS One* 2015; 10(10): e0139817. doi: 10.1371/journal.pone.0139817.

Simopoulos AP. An Increase in the Omega-6/Omega-3 Fatty Acid Ratio Increases the Risk for Obesity. *Nutrients* 2016; 8(3): 128. doi: 10.3390/nu8030128

Ye J. Mechanisms of insulin resistance in obesity. *Front Med* 2013; 7(1): 14–24. doi: 10.1007/s11684-013-0262-6

Osteoporosis

Barbagallo M, Dominguez L. Bone disorders associated with diabetes mellitus and its treatments. *Joint Bone Spine* 2019; 86(3): 315-320.

Choo MS, Choi SR, Han JH, Lee SH, Shim YS. Association of insulin resistance with near peak bone mass in the femur and lumbar spine of Korean adults aged 25-35: The Korean National Health and Nutrition Examination Survey 2008-2010. *PloS One* 13 July 2017. doi.org/10.1371/journal.pone.0177311

Gandhi SS, Muraresku C, McCormick EM, Falk MJ, McCormack SE. Risk factors for poor bone health in primary mitochondrial disease. *J Inherit Metab Dis* 2017; 40(5): 673-683. doi:10.1007/s10545-017-0046-2

Srikanthan P, Crandall CJ, Miller-Martinez D, et al. Insulin resistance and bone strength: findings from the study of midlife in the United States. *J Bone Miner Res* 2014; 29(4): 796-803. doi:10.1002/jbmr.2083

University of Pennsylvania. A link between mitochondrial damage and

osteoporosis. *Science Daily* 9 May 2019.
www.sciencedaily.com/releases/2019/05/190509153425.htm

Valderrabano RJ, Linares MI. Diabetes mellitus and bone health: epidemiology, etiology and implications for fracture risk stratification. *Clin Diabetes Endocrinol* 2018; 4: 9. doi: 10.1186/s40842-018-0060-9

Pancreas

Majumder S, Philip NA, Takahashi N, Levy MJ, Singh VP, Chari ST. Fatty Pancreas: Should We Be Concerned? *Pancreas* 2017; 46(10): 1251-1258. doi:10.1097/MPA.0000000000000941

Pothuraju R, Rachagani S, Junker WM, et al. Pancreatic cancer associated with obesity and diabetes: an alternative approach for its targeting. *J Exp Clin Cancer Res* 2018; 37: 319. doi: 10.1186/s13046-018-0963-4

Yu TY, Wang CYY. Impact of non–alcoholic fatty pancreas disease on glucose metabolism. *J Diabetes Investig* 2017; 8(6): 735–747. doi: 10.1111/jdi.12665

Pregnancy

Kahraman S, Dirice E, De Jesus DF, et al. Maternal insulin resistance and transient hyperglycemia impact the metabolic and endocrine phenotypes of offspring. *AJP: Endocrinology and Metabolism* 2014; 307 (10): E906. doi: 10.1152/ajpendo.00210.2014

Prostate problems

Di Sebastiano K M, Pinthus J H, Duivenvoorden WCM, Mourtzakis M. Glucose impairments and insulin resistance in prostate cancer: the role of obesity, nutrition and exercise. *Obes Rev* 2018; 19(7): 1008-1016. doi: 10.1111/obr.12674. Epub 2018 Mar 24.

Vikram A, Jena G, Ramarao P. Insulin-resistance and benign prostatic hyperplasia: the connection. *Eur J Pharmacol* 2010; 641(2-3): 75-81. doi:10.1016/j.ejphar.2010.05.042

Protein

Daley CA, Abbott A, Doyle PS, Nader GA, Larson S. A review of ftty acid profiles and antioxidant content in grass-fed and grain-fed beef. *Nutr J* 2010; 9: 10. 10. doi:10.1186/1475-2891-9-10

Karsten H, Patterson P, Stout R, Crews G. Vitamins A, E and fatty acid composition of the eggs of caged hens and pastured hens. *Renewable Agriculture and Food Systems* 2010; 25(1): 45-54. doi:10.1017/S1742170509990214

Layman DK, Anthony TG, Rasmussen BB, et al. Defining meal requirements for protein to optimize metabolic roles of amino acids. *Am J Clin Nutr* 2015; 101(6): 1330S–1338S. doi:10.3945/ajcn.114.084053

Leidy HJ, Clifton PM, Astrup A, et al. The role of protein in weight loss and maintenance. *Am J Clin Nutr* 2015; 101(6): 1320S–1329S. doi:10.3945/ajcn.114.084038

McAfee AJ, McSorley EM, Cuskelly GJ et al. Red meat from animals offered a grass diet increases plasma and platelet n-3 PUFA in healthy consumers. *Br J Nutr* 2011;105(1): 80-89. doi: 10.1017/S0007114510003090.

Zeraatkar D, Johnston BC, Bartoszko J, et al. Effect of Lower Versus Higher Red Meat Intake on Cardiometabolic and Cancer Outcomes: A Systematic Review of Randomized Trials. *Ann Intern Med* 2019; 10.7326/M19-0622. doi:10.7326/M19-0622

Zeraatkar D, Han MA, Guyatt GH, et al. Red and Processed Meat Consumption and Risk for All-Cause Mortality and Cardiometabolic Outcomes: A Systematic Review and Meta-analysis of Cohort Studies. *Ann Intern Med* 2019; 171: 703–710. doi.org/10.7326/M19-0655

Red meat and poultry

Daley CA, Abbott A., Doyle PS, et al. A review of fatty acid profiles and antioxidant content in grass-fed and grain-fed beef. *Nutr J* 2010; 9: 10. doi.org/10.1186/1475-2891-9-10

Jonhston BC, Zeraatkar D, Mi Ah Han, et al. Unprocessed Red Meat and Processed Meat Consumption: Dietary Guideline Recommendations From the Nutritional Recommendations

(NutriRECS) Consortium. *Annals of Internal Medicine* 2019; 171(10): 756-764

Kumar S, Sugihara F, Suzuki K, Inoue N, Venkateswarathirukumara S. A double-blind, placebo-controlled, randomised, clinical study on the effectiveness of collagen peptide on osteoarthritis. *J Sci Food Agric* 2015; 95(4): 702–707. doi:10.1002/jsfa.6752

Luo J, Yang Y, Liu J, et al. Systematic review with meta-analysis: meat consumption and the risk of hepatocellular carcinoma. *Aliment Pharmacol Ther* 2014; 39(9): 913–922. doi:10.1111/apt.12678

McAfee AJ, McSorley EM, Cuskelly GJ, et al. Red meat from animals offered a grass diet increases plasma and platelet n-3 PUFA in healthy consumers. *Br J Nutr* 2011; 105(1): 80–89. doi:10.1017/S0007114510003090

Mi Ah Han, Zeraatkar D, Guyatt G H et al. Reduction of Red and Processed Meat Intake and Cancer Mortality and Incidence. *Annals of Internal Medicine* 2019; 171(10): 711-720.

Ponnampalam EN, Mann NJ, Sinclair AJ. Effect of feeding systems on omega-3 fatty acids, conjugated linoleic acid and trans fatty acids in Australian beef cuts: potential impact on human health. *Asia Pac J Clin Nutr* 2006; 15(1): 21–29.

Ponte PI, Alves SP, Bessa RJ, et al. Influence of pasture intake on the fatty acid composition, and cholesterol, tocopherols, and tocotrienols content in meat from free-range broilers. *Poult Sci* 2008; 87(1): 80–88. doi:10.3382/ps.2007-00148

Turner ND, Lloyd SK. Association between red meat consumption and colon cancer: A systematic review of experimental results. *Experimental Biology and Medicine* 2019; 242(8): 813–839. doi.org/10.1177/1535370217693117

Zeraatkar D, Mi Ah Han, Guyatt GH, et al. Red and Processed Meat Consumption and Risk for All-Cause Mortality and Cardiometabolic Outcomes. *Annals of Internal Medicine* 2019; 171(10): 703-710.

Skin

Barth JH, Ng LL, Wojnarowska F, Dawber RP. Acanthosis nigricans, insulin resistance and cutaneous virilism. *Br J Dermatol* 1988: 118(5): 613-619.

Cheong HS, Chang Y, Joo EJ, Cho A, Ryu S. Metabolic Obesity Phenotypes and Risk of Cellulitis: A Cohort Study. *J Clin Med* 2019; 8(7): 953. doi:10.3390/jcm8070953

Gonzales-Saldivar G, Rodriguez-Gutierrez R, Ocampo-Candiani J, et al. Skin Manifestations of Insulin Resistance: From a Biochemical Stance to a Clinical Diagnosis and Management. *Dermatol Ther* 2017; 7(1): 37-51. doi: 10.1007/s13555-016-0160-3.

Mahmood SN, Bowe WP. Diet and Acne update: Carbohydrates Emerge as the Main Culprit. *J Drugs Dermatol* 2014; 13(4): 428-435.

Napolitano M, Megna M, Monfrecola G. Insulin Resistance and Skin Diseases. *Scientific World Journal* 2015; 2015: Article ID 479354. doi.org/10.1155/2015/479354

Shrestha P, Poudyal Y, Rajbhandari SL. Acrochordons and Diabetes Mellitus: A Case control Study. *Nepal Journal of Dermatology, Venereology & Leprology* 2015; 13(1): 32-37. doi.org/10.3126/njdvl.v13i1.14303

Sivakumar S, Banupriya K. A cross-sectional descriptive clinical study of dermatological manifestations in obesity. *International Journal of Research in Dermatology* 2017; 3(3): 2455-4529. doi.org/10.18203/issn.2455-4529.IntJResDermatol20173077

Sleep

Beccuti G, Pannain S. Sleep and obesity. *Curr Opin Clin Nutr Metab Care* 2011; 14(4): 402–412. doi: 10.1097/MCO.0b013e3283479109

Buxton OM. Sleep restriction for 1 week reduces insulin sensitivity in healthy men. *Diabetes* 2010; 59(9): 2126-2133.
http://diabetes.diabetesjournals.org/content/59/9/2126

Chaput JP, McNeil J, Després JP, Bouchard C, Tremblay A. Short sleep duration as a risk factor for the development of the metabolic syndrome in adults. *Prev Med* 2013; 57(6): 872–877.

Kim TW, Jeong J-H, Hong S-C. The Impact of Sleep and Circadian Disturbance on Hormones and Metabolism. *International Journal of Endocrinology* 2015; 2015: Article ID 591729. doi.org/10.1155/2015/591729

Knutson KL, Spiegel K, Penev P, Van Cauter E. The metabolic consequences of sleep deprivation. *Sleep Med Rev* 2007; 11(3): 163–178.

Morselli L, Leproult R, Balbo M, Spiegel K. Role of sleep duration in the regulation of glucose metabolism and appetite. Best practice & research. *Clinical Endocrinology & Metabolism* 2010; 24(5): 687–702. doi.org/10.1016/j.beem.2010.07.005

Owino S, Buonfiglio DDC, Tchio C, Tosini G. Melatonin Signaling a Key Regulator of Glucose Homeostasis and Energy Metabolism. *Front Endocrinol* 2019. doi.org/10.3389/fendo.2019.00488

Poroyko VA, Carreras A, Khalyfa A, et al. Chronic Sleep Disruption Alters Gut Microbiota, Induces Systemic and Adipose Tissue Inflammation and Insulin Resistance in Mice. *Sci Rep* 2016; 6: 35405. doi.org/10.1038/srep35405

Reutrakul S, Van Cauter E. Interactions between sleep, circadian function, and glucose metabolism: Implications for risk and severity of diabetes. *Ann N Y Acad Sci* 2014; 1311: 151-173. doi: 10.1111/nyas.12355.

Sleep apnoea and snoring

Almendros I, Garcia-Rio F. Sleep apnoea, insulin resistance and diabetes: the first step is in the fat. *European Respiratory Journal* 2017; 49: 1700179. doi: 10.1183/13993003.00179-2017

Ip MS, Lam B, Ng MM, et al.Obstructive Sleep Apnea Is Independently Associated with Insulin Resistance. *Am J Respir Crit Care Med* 2002; 165(5): 670-676.

Siegmann MJ, Athinarayanan SJ, Hallberg SJ, et al.Improvement in patient-reported sleep in type 2 diabetes and prediabetes participants receiving a continuous care intervention with nutritional ketosis. *Sleep Medicine* 2019; 55: 92-99.

Zhu J, Song F, Xu H, et al. The Relationship between Simple Snoring and Metabolic Syndrome: A Cross-Sectional Study. *Journal of Diabetes Research* 2019; 2019: Article ID 9578391. doi.org/10.1155/2019/9578391

Smoking

Ballweg K, Mutze K, Königshoff M, Eickelberg O, Meiners S. Cigarette smoke extract affects mitochondrial function in alveolar epithelial cells. *Am J Physiol Lung Cell Mol Physiol* 2014; 307(11): L895-L907.

doi:10.1152/ajplung.00180.2014

Pourahmad J, Aghvami M, Zarei MH, Naserzadeh P. Cigarette Smoke and Mitochondrial Damage. In: Dykens W, Dykens JA (eds). *Mitochondrial Dysfunction Caused by Drugs and Environmental Toxicants*. Chichester: Wiley; 2018; pp 709-725. doi:10.1002/9781119329725.ch45

Smoking and Inflammation. *PLoS Medicine* 2005; 2(6): e198. https://doi.org/10.1371/journal.pmed.0020198

Steptoe A, Ussher M. Smoking, cortisol and nicotine. *Int J Psychophysiol* 2006; 59(3): 228-235. doi:10.1016/j.ijpsycho.2005.10.011

Sweeteners

Murray S, Tulloch A, Criscitelli K, Avena NM. Recent Studies of the Effects of Sugars on Brain Systems Involved in Energy Balance and Reward: Relevance to Low Calorie Sweeteners. *Physiol Behav* 2016; 164(Pt B): 504–508. doi: 10.1016/j.physbeh.2016.04.004

Pepino MY, Tiemann CD, Patterson BW, Wice BM, Klein S. Sucralose affects glycemic and hormonal responses to an oral glucose load. *Diabetes Care* 2013; 36(9): 2530-2535. doi: 10.2337/dc12-2221.

Yang Q. Gain weight by "going diet?" Artificial sweeteners and the neurobiology of sugar cravings. *Yale J Biol Med* 2010; 83(2): 101–108.

Thyroid, POCS, endocrine system

Bailey B, Phinney S, Volek J. Polycystic Ovarian Syndrome, Insulin Resistance, and Inflammation. *Virta Health* 15 Jan 2019. www.virtahealth.com/blog/pcos-polycystic-ovarian-syndrome

Hutchins J. Your Blood Sugar May Be the Key to Your Hormone Imbalance. *Diabetes & Endocrinology* 11 November 2015. https://health.clevelandclinic.org/polycystic-ovary-syndrome-pill-not-remedy/

Kulshreshtha B, Arpita A, Rajesh PT, et al. Adolescent gynecomastia is associated with a high incidence of obesity, dysglycemia, and family background of diabetes mellitus. *Indian J Endocrinol Metab* 2017; 21(1): 160–164. doi: 10.4103/2230-8210.196022

Marshall JC, Dunaif. All Women With PCOS Should Be Treated For

The evidence

Insulin Resistance. *Fertil Steril* 2012; 97(1): 18–22. doi: 10.1016/j.fertnstert.2011.11.036

NHS. Causes: Polycystic ovary syndrome – Causes. www.nhs.uk/conditions/polycystic-ovary-syndrome-pcos/causes/ (30 June 2020)

Peppa M, Koliaki C, et al. Skeletal Muscle Insulin Resistance in Endocrine Disease. *J Biomed Bio-technol* 2010; 2010: 527850.

Robeva R, Elenkova A, Zacharieva S. Causes and Metabolic Consequences of Gynecomastia in Adult Patients. *International Journal of Endocrinology* 2019; 2019: Article ID 6718761. doi.org/10.1155/2019/6718761

Rogowicz-Frontczak A, Majchrzak A, Zozulińska-Ziółkiewicz D. Insulin resistance in endocrine disorders – treatment options. *Endokrynol Pol* 2017; 68(3): 334-351. doi: 10.5603/EP.2017.0026.

Vyakaranam S, Vanaparthy S, Nori S, Palarapu S, Bhongir AV. Study of Insulin Resistance in Subclinical Hypothyroidism. *International Journal of Health Sciences and Research* 2014; 4(9): 147–153.

Williams G. Aromatase up-regulation, insulin and raised intracellular oestrogens in men, induce adiposity, metabolic syndrome and prostate disease, via aberrant ER-α and GPER signalling. *Mol Cell Endocrinol* 2012; 351(2): 269–278. doi:10.1016/j.mce.2011.12.017

Index

acanthosis nigricans 40
addictions 111–112
additives, avoiding 98
adrenal disorders 52
adrenaline 23, 37, 105
advanced glycation end products (AGEs) 18–19, 67, 76
aging
    Alzheimer's disease and 66
    cell damage and 11 12
    low-carb diet and 76
    macular degeneration relating to 69
    mitochondrial function and 12
    muscle mass and 84, 89
alcohol 19–20, 107
aldehydes and refined oils 21, 22
alpha-linolenic acid (ALA) 20, 95
Alzheimer's disease 66–68, 69
    references 177–178
amino acids
    essential 1, 2, 88
    in free-range meat and poultry 91, 91–92
angiogenesis, cancer 65
antibiotics 99
anti-inflammatory factors 21, 29
antioxidants 86, 87, 88, 95
    references 177
anxiety 103, 104, 105, 106
apoptosis 9, 85
ashwagandha 104
atherosclerosis 11, 62

aubergine parmigiana 154
autoimmune illnesses/diseases 28, 34, 52, 56, 75, 80
autonomic neuropathy 35, 177–178
autophagy 9, 12, 83, 84

bacteria
    in gut *see* microbiome
    probiotic 96, 97
beans, high carb content 156
beef
    goulash, with celeriac mash 153
    stuffed peppers filled with 151
beer 20
belly (deep) breathing 105–106
berries 82, 88, 155, 156
    references 188
beta cells, pancreatic. 3, 19
blood-brain barrier 67
blood glucose *see* sugar
blood pressure, raised (hypertension) 41–42, 109
    medication for 111
bowel problems 54–55
    see also gut
brain 66–69, 103
    foggy 36
    gut–brain axis 27, 57, 99, 102
    see also mental health; mind
bread 18, 79, 111
breakfast 117–118
    carb-loaded 18
    leaving out 84

breast enlargement, men 52–53
breathing, deep 105–106
broccoli
    grilled cod with red salsa and tenderstem broccoli 148
    in kale-onion-goats' cheese pie 125
    leek and broccoli soup 120
    in other dishes 125, 126, 141, 146

cabbage 118, 155
    fermented *see* sauerkraut
calcium and smoking 31
calories 112
cancer xi-xii, 63–66
    references 181–182
carbohydrates (dietary) 1–2
    diet low in *see* low-carbohydrate diet
    excess 33, 44, 49, 50, 112
    foods and their content of 155–156
    and sugars converted to/stored as fat 2, 3, 47, 49, 77
    see also sugar (dietary)
cardiac problems *see* heart
carnosine 91
carrageenan 99
cauliflower
    pork and pepper stew with cauliflower rice 147
    shepherd's pie with 142–143
celeriac mash, beef goulash with 153
cell(s)
    autophagy 9, 12, 83, 84
    cancer, growth and development 64–66
    development of insulin resistance 34
    programmed cell death 9, 85
cereals grains *see* grains
cheese (in recipes)
    dinner 134, 139, 140, 142, 143, 144, 145, 149, 151, 154
    lunch 124, 126, 127, 128, 130, 131
    soups 120, 123
chicken
    and coconut soup 119
    one-pan chicken and vegetables 141

children and young people/teenagers 114–115
    overweight/obese 48, 114
    sugar consumption 17
chilli con carne 144
cholesterol 42–44
    'bad' 42, 43
    'good' 42, 43
    heart disease and 62–63
    references 189–190
choline 91
chronic fatigue syndrome 57
chronic illness and symptoms xi, xiii, xiv, 33
    genes and 16
    prevention and reduction 22
    stress and 23
chronic inflammation *see* inflammation
chronic pain 56–57, 182–183
chronic stress 23–24, 30, 39, 99, 106
coconut soups
    chicken and 119
    fish and 122
cod
    casserole, with mushrooms 139
    grilled, with red salsa and tenderstem broccoli 148
coeliac disease 80
coenzyme Q10 91, 92
coffee 81, 85, 90, 104, 118
colitis, ulcerative 54
constipation 54, 55
    with low-carbohydrate diet 109
coronary heart disease *see* heart disease
cortisol 23, 24, 25, 27, 29, 30, 52, 60, 105
cost of healthy diet 118
courgette and smoked fish cakes 131
cravings for food 37, 47, 76, 77, 78, 111–112
cream 90
cream sauce (and creamy sauce) 146
    sage and 138
Crohn's disease 54

dairy 90
    carbohydrate content 155, 156

Index

deep breathing 105–106
dementia 66–68
dental problems *see* oral and dental problems
depression 68, 102, 103, 104
DHA (docosahexaenoic acid) 20, 21, 92, 95
diabetes
    cancer and 64
    complications 19
        retinopathy 19, 69
    infection predisposition 40
    low-carb diet in treatment of 61
    medication and 111
    maternal/gestational 48, 113–114
diabetes type 1 85, 111
diabetes type 2 59–62, 84
    diagnosis 34
    mitochondria and 10
    references 183–184
diabetes type 3 66, 69
diabetes type 4 69
diagnosing insulin resistance 33–45
diaphragmatic (deep) breathing 105–106
diet (and nutrition) xv
    cost of healthy diet 118
    diabetes treated via 61
    gut microbiome and 28, 95
    ketogenic 75, 84, 85
    low-carbohydrate *see* low-carbohydrate diet
    in reversal of insulin resistance 72, 74–100, 103–104, 117–118
    see also eating too often; food; meals; supplements
digestive tract *see* gut
dill-lemon sauce 131
dinner 134–154
    intermittent fasting and 54
    recipes 134–154
disaccharides 16
DNA xvi
docosahexaenoic acid (DHA) 20, 21, 92, 95
dressing for goats' cheese and bacon salad 127
drinks 80–82
drugs *see* medications

e-cigarettes 31
ear problems, inner 40–41, 192
eating too often 7, 12, 22–23, 37, 82–85
    see also diet; food; meals
eggs 92
    Mediterranean 132
eicosanoids 21
eicosapentaenoic acid (EPA) 20, 21, 92, 95, 104
electrolyte balance, insulin effects 5
endocrine system *see* hormones
endometriosis 53, 53–54
energy levels, low 12–13, 36–37, 37
EPA (eicosapentaenoic acid) 20, 21, 92, 95, 104
epigenetics xvi, 48
essential oils 106
exercise 29–30, 99, 100–102
    bedtime and 107
    intensive (HIIT) 100–102
    ketones and 76
    lack of 29–30
    mental health and 102, 105
    references 186–187
eye problems 68
    references 188

fasting
    insulin levels 35
    intermittent 61, 83–85
fat (body), visceral 7
fat (dietary - lipid and oils) 2–3, 90, 94–95
    heart disease and 43, 44, 62–63
    insulin effects on metabolism 5
    low-fat diets 90
    natural fats 94–95, 155
    references 184–185
    refined oils 20–22, 94–95
    sugars and carbohydrates converted to/stored as 2, 3, 47, 49, 77
fatigue *see* chronic fatigue syndrome; tiredness
fatty acids
    essential 1, 74, 90, 94
    monounsaturated 20, 22, 95
    omega-3 *see* omega-3 fatty acids
    omega-6 20, 21, 95

omega-7 20
polyunsaturated fats (PUFAs) 20, 95
references 184–185
saturated (SFAs) 20, 22, 62, 63, 94, 95
sources 3
fatty fish 92, 95
fatty liver 49–51
　alcoholic 19
　non-alcoholic (NAFLD) xii, 17, 49–51, 77
　references 187–188
fatty pancreas 51
fermented products/foods 90, 96–97
　soy 92, 155
fibre 80, 87, 91, 110
　references 189
　soluble 97
fibromyalgia xi, 56–57
fight-or-flight response 24
fish 92
　fatty 92, 95
　recipes 122, 129, 130, 131, 139, 140, 145, 146, 148, 152
fluid retention 41, 109
FODMAPs 98
foetus, hyperinsulinaemia 113–114
food(s)
　additives 98
　carbohydrate content 155–156
　craving 37, 47, 76, 77, 78, 111–112
　eating too often 7, 12, 22–23, 37, 82–85
　fermented see fermented products
　good quality real 85–86, 90, 94, 104
　　children/teenagers 114
　see also diet; meals and recipes; supplements
free-range meat 90, 91, 94
frittata, vegetable 126
fructose (fruit sugar) 2, 16–17, 19, 50, 78
　cancer and 64
　gut health and 98
　uric acid levels and 59
fruit 87–88

medium and high carbohydrate content 156
references 188
fruit sugar see fructose

GABA (gamma-aminobutyric acid) 27
galactose 2, 16
gamma-aminobutyric acid (GABA) 27
gardening 101
garlic
　oven-roasted salmon with 146
　spaghetti squash with garlic mushrooms 134–135
gastrointestinal tract see gut
gastroparesis 55
genes and chronic illness 16
gestational diabetes 48, 113–114
ghrelin 3, 24
glaucoma 68
　references 188
GLP-1 27–28
glucagon 3, 4, 6, 23, 27, 47–48, 60, 75, 82
glucagon-like peptide 1 (GLP-1) 27–28
glucose
　blood see sugar (blood)
　in brain, high levels 67
　eating and 3
　glycogen breakdown into (glycogenolysis) 8, 84
　in liver, manufacture (gluconeogenesis) 7–8, 49, 89
　stored as fat 3, 47
　stored as glycogen 3, 16, 17, 29, 49
glutathione 91
gluten sensitivity 80, 98
glycation, end products of (AGEs) 18–19, 67, 76
glycine 91–92
glycogen 4
　breaking down into glucose (glycogenolysis) 8, 84
　fructose stored as 2
　glucose stored as 3, 16, 17, 29, 49
goats' cheese
　bacon salad with 127
　kale-onion-goats' cheese pie 125

Index

spinach soup with 123
gout 58–59
    references 188–189
grains
    avoidance 79–80
    high-carb content 79, 156
Greek meatballs and tzatziki sauce 136–137
Greek salad 128
green tea 104–105
growth hormone 64, 84
    exercise and 100
gut (digestive/gastrointestinal system)
    brain–gut axis 27, 57, 99, 102
    exercise and 30
    healthy (healthy bowel) 28, 95–100
        references 178–181
    leaky gut syndrome 28, 30, 54, 96, 97
    microbiome *see* microbiome
    see also bowel problems; stomach problems
gynaecomastia 52–53

haddock gratin, smoked 145
haemoglobin A1C (HbA1C) 19, 61
HbA1C 19, 61
HDL (high density lipoprotein) 31, 42–44, 62
heart disease (coronary) 34, 62–63
    blood pressure and 41
    lipids (LDL/cholesterol/triglycerides) and 43, 44, 62–63
    references 189–190
heart palpitations and low-carb diets 110
herbs 86
    teas made from 85, 118
high density lipoprotein (HDL) 31, 42–44, 62
high intensity interval training (HIIT) 100–102
hiking 101
hippocampus 67
Hippocrates xv
hormones (and endocrine system) 3

eating too often and 12, 22
gut health and 27–28
insulin effects on other hormones 5
menopause and 115–116
mitochondrial function and 11–12
polycystic ovarian syndrome and 53–55
references 204–205
sleep and 24–25
smoking and 31
stress hormones 23, 24, 27, 29, 100, 105
hygiene
    oral 53
    sleep 107
hypercholesterolaemia 63
hyperglycaemia (high blood sugar/glucose) 15, 36, 59, 61, 111
    advanced glycation end products formation in 18–19
hyperinsulinaemia 6–8, 15, 31, 34, 39, 64
    adverse effects 33, 51, 109
    in pregnancy 112–114
    insulin use adding to problem of 61
hypertension *see* blood pressure
hypoglycaemia (low blood glucose/sugar) 35, 36–37
hypothalamus 68

IGFs (insulin-like growth factors) 39, 64
immune system 37–38
    chronic inflammation and 10
    exercise and 30
    gut microbiome and 27, 38
    insulin and 3, 38, 39, 76
    references 191
    stress and 24
infections
    diabetes-related predisposition to 40
    recurrent acute 37–38
inflammation (chronic) 10–13, 38, 44
    anti-inflammatory factors 21, 29
    autoimmunity/coeliac disease and 80

brain/neurological problems and 67, 68
cancer and 64
eye disease and 68
fatty liver disease and 49
immune dysfunction and 38
preventing/reducing 22, 44, 74, 92
pro-inflammatory factors 10, 21
references 191–192
smoking and 31
inflammatory bowel disease (IBD) 54, 55, 58
inflammatory skin conditions 40
inner ear problems 40–41, 192
insulin 3–6, 23
brain function and 67
excess (in blood) *see* hyperinsulinaemia
fasting levels 35
functions 4–5
immunity and 3, 38, 39, 76
spikes (in production) 77, 79, 81, 88
therapeutic use 62
insulin-like growth factors (IGFs) 39, 64
insulin resistance
causes 15–32, 33
references 158–161
consequences 47–70
references 161–165
defining 1–13
references 157–158
effects 4–5
reversing 71–107, 110, 112, 117–118
children/teenagers 114
diet 72, 74–100, 103–104, 117–118
key actions 73–107
references 165–175
signs and symptoms (and diagnosis) 35–45
references 161
special considerations 109–116
references 175–176
insulin sensitivity
exercise effects on 29

pregnancy and 112–113
internal ear problems 40–41, 192
irritable bowel syndrome (IBS) 54, 56, 98

juices and smoothies 81–82, 117–118

ketogenic diet 75, 84, 85
kidney function 41, 109

lactofermentation 96
lactose 2, 16, 81, 90, 98, 118
LDL (low density lipoprotein) 42–44, 62
leaky gut syndrome 28, 30, 54, 96, 97
leek and broccoli soup 120
legumes, high carb content 156
leptin 3, 24
lifestyle factors/problems (and interventions/changes/measures) 12, 15, 29, 57, 73, 77, 109, 110
type 2 diabetes 59, 60, 61
linoleic acid (LA) 21
α- linolenic acid (alpha-linolenic acid; ALA) 20, 95
lipid *see* fat
lipoprotein
high density (HDL) 31, 42–44, 62
low density (LDL) 42–44, 62
liver 48–51, 60
alcohol-related problems 19
carbohydrate excess and 33, 44, 49, 50
diabetes type 2 and 60
fatty *see* fatty liver
fructose metabolism 17
glucose manufacture (gluconeogenesis) 7–8, 49, 89
immune system and 38–39
pan-fried, with sage and cream sauce 138
low-carbohydrate diet 61–62, 74–77, 82, 85, 87, 109, 109–111
addictions and 111–112
benefits 74–77
food and dietary regime for 78–79, 80, 83, 88, 90, 93, 97–98, 155

Index

intensive exercise and 100, 101
mental health and 103, 105
problems 109–111
references 192–195
sugar-free 64, 98
water 81
low density lipoprotein (LDL) 42–44, 62
low-fat diets 90
lunch 124–133
   intermittent fasting and 54
   lunch box foods 93
   recipes 124–133

mackerel 93
   smoked mackerel salad 129
macular degeneration, age-related 68
magnesium 110
   supplements 86
Malhotra, Aseem 63
maltose 2, 16
margarines 94
meals and recipes 117–154
meat
   free-range 91–92
   recipes 136–138, 141–144, 147, 151, 153
   references 200–201
meatballs, Greek, and tzatziki sauce 136–137
medications (drugs) 12, 71–72
   glucose level-controlling 60–62
   low-carb diets and 111
   side effects 71
   vitamin B12 absorption affected by 58
meditation 105–106
Mediterranean eggs 132
melatonin 24, 25, 26, 27, 106
memory problems 36–37, 67–68
menopause 115–116
mental health (psychological) problems/symptoms 102–106
   exercise and 102, 105
   gut microbiome and 27
   see also anxiety; depression; mind; stress
metabolic syndrome 8, 28, 41, 43
   bowel problems and 54

gout and 58
metabolism 1–3
metastases 65
microbiome/flora, gut (balances/imbalances) 26–28, 57
   coeliac disease and 80
   diet and 28, 96
   exercise and 30
   fibromyalgia and 56–57
   immunity and 27, 38
   mouth 53
   neurological problems and 68
   references 178–181
   sleep problems and 25
micronutrients 85–86, 87, 91, 92, 104, 114, 177
   in berries 88
   in eggs 92
   mitochondrial function and 10
   supplements 86
milk 81, 90
mind 72–73, 102, 103, 105
   see also mental health
mindfulness 105, 106
mitochondria 8–10
   damage/dysfunction 10, 11, 12–13, 15, 18, 27, 29, 31, 37, 196–197
   brain/neurological problems and 68
   cancer and 65
   glaucoma and 79
   medications associated with 71–72
   osteoporosis and 54
   pregnancy and 113
   low-carb diet and 76
   references 196–197
monosaccharides 16
monounsaturated fatty acids 20, 22, 95
mouth *see* oral and dental problems
mozzarella, baked portobello mushrooms with peppers and pesto and 149–150
muscle mass 5, 29, 84, 89
   references 197
mushrooms
   baked portobello, with mozzarella

and peppers and pesto 149–150
cod casserole with 139
garlic, spaghetti-style squash and 134–135

nervous system disorders *see* neurological problems; neuropathy
neurological problems 66–68
neuropathy
   autonomic 35, 177–178
   peripheral 57–58
neurotransmitters 27
nutrition *see* diet; eating too often; food; meals; supplements
nuts and seeds 90
   low-carbohydrate 155
   medium- and high-carbohydrate 156
   seed oils 21–22

obesity and overweight/excess weight 36, 47–48, 72
   children/young people 48, 114
   gout and 58
   references 196–197
   sleep apnoea and 39
oestrogen
   dominance 52, 115
   menopause and 115, 116
oils *see* essential oils; fat (dietary)
oligosaccharides, prebiotic 97
olive oil and oleic acid 22, 91, 95
omega-3 fatty acids 20–21, 21, 90, 91, 92, 94, 95, 96, 98
   supplements 104
omega-6 fatty acids 20, 21, 95
omega-9 fatty acids 20
onion-kale-goats' cheese pie 125
oral and dental problems 53
   references 183
organ meat 91
organic foods 85, 88, 94
osteoporosis 31, 54
   references 198–199
outdoor exercise 101, 105
ovaries and polycystic ovarian syndrome (POCS) 53–55, 204–205
overweight *see* obesity and overweight
oxidative stress 10, 11, 29, 31, 68, 69, 76, 85, 88, 113

pain, chronic 56–57, 182–183
pancreas 3, 7, 34
   fatty 51
   inflammation (pancreatitis) 44
   pregnancy and 113, 114
   references 199
peppers
   baked portobello mushrooms with mozzarella and pesto and 149–150
   pork and pepper stew with cauliflower rice 147
   stuffed, with beef filling 151
peripheral neuropathy 57–58
pernicious anaemia 58
pesticides 93
pesto, baked portobello mushrooms with mozzarella and peppers and 149–150
physical exercise *see* exercise
placenta 113–114
polycystic ovarian syndrome (PCOS) 53–55, 204–205
pork and pepper stew with cauliflower rice 147
portobello mushrooms (baked) with mozzarella and peppers and pesto 149–150
poultry
   free-range 91–92
   recipes 119, 141
   references 200–201
prebiotics 96, 97–98
pre-diabetes 59
pregnancy 48, 112–114
   references 199
probiotics 96–97
   references 177
processed (refined) foods 92–94
   meat 92
   oils 20–22, 94–95
progesterone 52, 94, 115

Index

programmed cell death 9, 85
pro-inflammatory factors 10, 21
prostate problems 52
   references 199–200
proteins 2, 88–92
   amounts to eat 89–90
   references 200
   sources 90–92
psychological problems *see* mental health problems
pumpkin soup 121

quiche (homemade) 124

reactive oxygen species 11, 76
recipes and meals 117–154
refined foods *see* processed foods
relaxation 102, 106
renal (kidney) function 41, 109
retinopathy (diabetic) 19, 69
   references 188
root (below ground) vegetables 79, 87, 88, 156

sage and cream sauce 138
salads 127–129
salmon
   baked, and spinach 130
   oven-roasted, with garlic 146
salt and sodium 109–111
saturated fats (SFAs) 20, 22, 62, 63, 94, 95
sauces 154
   cream *see* cream sauce
   dill-lemon 131
   tzatziki 137
sauerkraut 96
   easy (recipe) 133
seeds *see* nuts and seeds
serotonin 27, 30, 105
sex hormones and menopause 115–116
shepherd's pie with cauliflower 142–143
signs and symptoms
   insulin resistance *see* insulin resistance
   mitochondrial dysfunction or damage 12–13

skin conditions 39–40
   references 201
sleep 44–45, 106–107
   references 202–203
sleep apnoea 39, 75, 106, 107
   references 203
smoking 30–31
   references 203
smoothies and juices 81–82, 117–118
snoring 39, 75, 106, 107
   references 203
sodium and salt 109–111
soups 119–123
soy, fermented 92, 155
spaghetti squash with garlic mushrooms 134–135
spinach
   baked salmon and 130, 130
   oven-roasted salmon with garlic 146
   soup 123
squash (spaghetti-style) and garlic mushrooms 134–135
starch/starchy foods 2
   avoidance 78–79
stomach problems 55
stress 23–24, 102–106
   chronic 23–24, 30, 39, 99, 106
   hormones of 23, 24, 27, 29, 100, 105
   management 24, 99, 102–106
sucrose 16
sugar (blood sugar/blood glucose) 16
   body's loss of control 34
   cancer and 64, 65
   and carbs converted to/stored as fat 2, 3, 47, 49, 77
   controlling our levels of 60–62
   high *see* hyperglycaemia
   insulin and 3, 4, 6, 7
   low (hypoglycaemia) 35, 36–37
sugar (dietary sugars) xiii, xiv, 1–2, 16–17, 16–18
   advice and recommendations 18, 186
   cutting out 77–82
   low-carbohydrate diet without 64, 98
   stored as fat 23

sugar (table) 16
supplements 104
    micronutrients 86
sweeteners
    artificial 78
        references 204
    'natural' 77
    sugar-like 17, 19, 77–78
symptoms *see* signs and symptoms

T-cells 30
tea 81, 85, 104, 118
    green 104–105
    herbal 85, 118
teenagers *see* children and young people/teenagers
teeth *see* oral and dental problems
testosterone 51, 63, 94, 115
thyroid dysfunction 52
tinnitus 40–41
tiredness 12–13, 25, 37
tooth problems *see* oral and dental problems
toxic digestive metabolites 28
triglycerides 17, 42–43
    elevated/high/raised blood levels 31, 36, 43, 44, 50
tuna bake 140
tzatziki sauce 137

ulcerative colitis 54
ultra-processed foods 93
United States (US) xii
uric acid levels 58–59
US xii

vaping 31
vegetable(s) 79, 80, 86
    carbohydrate content 155, 156
    cost 118
    fermented 96–97
    in juices and smoothies 81–82
    references 188
    root (below ground) 79, 87, 88, 156
vegetable frittata 126
vegetable oils 10, 21, 22, 99
visceral fat 7
vitamin B12 58, 91, 92
    deficiency 58, 60
vitamin C 86
vitamin D (and D3) 86
    smoking and 31

waistline, expanding 36
walking 101
water with low-carbohydrate diet 81
weight
    gaining 7, 36, 47, 50
        see also obesity
    losing 47, 75, 112
working memory problems 36–37

yoga 102
young people *see* children and young people

Also from Hammersmith Health Books…

Conquer Type 2 Diabetes

How a fat, middle-aged man lost 31 kilos and reversed his type 2 diabetes

By Richard Shaw

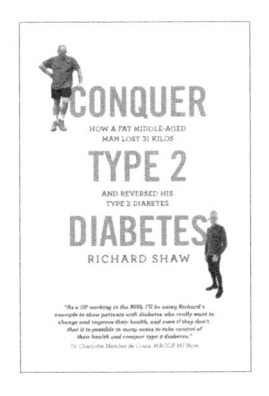

Type-2 diabetes doesn't have to be a lifelong condition; for many people, especially those who have been recently diagnosed, it's possible to reverse the symptoms of this malignant disease. But how can that be done? In 2017 the author, inspired by results obtained from research done at Newcastle University, UK, decided to try and kick the disease by following a carefully structured, low-carb, whole-food diet and starting a modest exercise regime. *Conquer Type 2 Diabetes* describes what he did to lose 31 kilos and all his diabetes signs (high blood sugar, high cholesterol, high blood pressure) and symptoms.

www.hammersmithbooks.co.uk/product/conquer-type-2-diabetes/

Also from Hammersmith Health Books...

Prevent and Cure Diabetes

Delicious diets, not dangerous drugs

By Dr Sarah Myhill

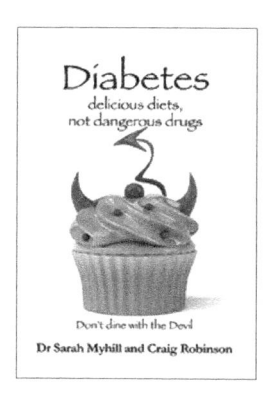

As Dr Myhill writes: 'All medical therapies start with diet. Modern Western diets are driving modern epidemics of diabetes, heart disease, cancer and dementia; this process is called metabolic syndrome. In this book I explain in detail why and how we have arrived at a situation where the real weapons of mass destruction can be found in our kitchens. Importantly, the book describes the vital steps every one of us can make to reverse the situation so that life can be lived to its full potential.'

**www.hammersmithbooks.co.uk/product/
prevent-cure-diabetes/**